*"We can easily forgive a child who is afraid of the dark;
the real tragedy of life is when adults are afraid of the light."*

— PLATO

My mother died the moment I was born, and so for my whole life there was nothing standing between myself and eternity; at my back was always a bleak, black wind. I could not have known at the beginning of my life that this would be so; I only came to know this in the middle of my life, just at the time when I was no longer young and realized that I had less of some of the things I used to have in abundance and more of some of the things I scarcely had at all. And this realization of loss and gain made me look backward and forward: at my beginning was this woman whose face I had never seen, but at my end was nothing, no one between me and the black room of the world. I came to feel that for my whole life I had been standing on a precipice, that my loss had made me vulnerable, hard, and helpless; on knowing this I became overwhelmed with sadness and shame and pity for myself.

— JAMAICA KINCAID, *The Autobiography of My Mother*

AFRAID OF THE DAY

afraid of the day

a daughter's journey

NANCY GRAHAM

WOMEN'S PRESS · TORONTO

Afraid of the Day: A Daughter's Journey
First published in 2003 by
Women's Press, an imprint of Canadian Scholars' Press Inc.
180 Bloor Street West, Suite 801
Toronto, Ontario
M5S 2V6
www.womenspress.ca

Canadian Scholars' Press / Women's Press gratefully acknowledges financial support for our publishing activities from the Ontario Arts Council, the Canada Council for the Arts, the Government of Canada through the Book Publishing Industry Development Program (BPIDP), and the Government of Ontario through the Ontario Book Publishers Tax Credit Program and through the Ontario Book Initiative.

For various reasons, some names have been changed.

National Library of Canada Cataloguing in Publication Data
Graham, Nancy, 1962–
   Afraid of the day : a daughter's journey / Nancy Graham.
ISBN 0-88961-413-X
1. Graham, Nancy, 1962—Family.   2. Children of depressed persons.
3. Depressed persons—Family relationships.   I. Title.
RC537.G73 2003   362.2'5   C2003-901535-1

Cover and text design by George Kirkpatrick
Cover photo by Jolie Dobson
Author photo by Kenna Park

03   04   05   06   07   08   6   5   4   3   2   1

Printed and bound in Canada by AGMV Marquis Imprimeur Inc.

For my Mom, in trying to make sense of it all ...

Contents

Acknowledgements

THROUGHOUT THE writing of this book, during the formative years beforehand, and in the journey ever since, I have been blessed with a richly textured life, through which a tapestry of souls have offered their support, friendship, and guidance in one way or another.

June Callwood, to whom destiny guided me back in 1996, by virtue of the North York Public Library's Writer-in-Residence Program. Your inspiration and encouragement over the years fuelled my determination to break through the web of depression with words. Thank you for sharing of yourself as you have.

To the staff at Canadian Scholars' Press/Women's Press, for your confidence in this work and for the effort you have all put into it. In particular, Althea Prince, Managing Editor: I hope I have done you proud by proving to be an author who "walks good" and is not "afraid of the day." And Rebecca Conolly, for your enthusiasm and your soulful, sensitive copyediting.

With enormous gratitude to the following five readers, for their willingness and honesty: Sharon Day, whose sisterly heart and soul have blessed my life since childhood; Pam Mountain, whose friendship emerged as the silver lining in the darkest of caves; Ellen Pente, for your trust when I came out of the woodwork; Helen McLean, who generously showed this novice a thing or two about skiing; and Jean Kowalewski, for finding the title between the light of Plato and the puddles of Woolf, and for everything else amber between the lines, "dziekuje."

With thanks to Marie Robertson, for getting me to "write down the bones," as if I had only six months to live; and nine years later, to Bernadette Dyer, who extended an author's hand behind her during the last months before publication.

Where would I be now, on the other side of 40, without steadfast good friends of old and new: Elaine (Honda) Ryoji, Kim (Ramsay) Kup, Peigi Ross, Susan (Hamouda) Julian, Jenny Hughes, Danielle (VanderVliet) Lloyd, Lori McCall, Wendy (Russ) Norris, Leanne Elliott, Mimi Shea, Manon Duguay, SilviaWannam, Barbara Ades, and Donna King. And to Theo Heras, for whom singing is the life blood and life breath that writing is to me.

With blessings for inner peace, to other friends who have variously shared what it's like to be afraid of the day: Josephine Vaccaro-Chang, Diane Corbeil-Thomson, Claire Fyfe, Marina Bourikas, and Barbara Center. And to Kathy Crouch, I hope this book reaches you.

During those years of my Mom's illness when nothing made sense, and in the aftermath of her relative wellness, I am grateful beyond words to my aunts and uncles, Doris and John Grist, Bev and Allan Graham; to neighbours Irene Karl and Eleanor Towers; to my mother's lifelong friend, Lillian Bottrill. Thank you for offering safe havens and for sharing your recollections as candidly as you did. I also acknowledge Kay Honda, for her perspective on then and now, and to Ruth Chasty and Dorothy Elliott for your unflinching friendship with my Mom through the years.

I would further like to acknowledge this book was written in memory of Elsie and Albert Hulls, and Robina and Henry Graham, Lillian and Larry Smith, Grace and Bob Hubbard, Anne and George Bonner, Jack Grist and Bruce Towers, all who left this world never knowing Mom in her relative wellness. And for Madge and Casey Harrison, Betty Grist and Edith Inman, who did. And for my dear departed centenarian Sunset neighbour Impi Nurmi: it's finally published!

I would be remiss if I did not acknowledge my Toronto Public Library colleagues, for a better workplace this writer could not have.

To the extraordinary women of the Jean Tweed Centre, specifically Virginia Ross, Lynne Macdonell, Nanci Harris, and Carol Garry, for keeping me grounded in my recovered and rediscovered life.

And to Dr. Hannah Wilansky, for navigating me through the turbulent waters, up over the vast expanse of weather-beaten rock, allowing me unconditional opportunity to untangle decades of knots and to ultimately find freedom.

Thank you Steven, Mom, and Dad, because I know this can't be easy.

For being there for my little brother through his own rites of passage, I thank Dawnna.

To my beloved canine companions: dearly departed C.C., who comforted me through many raw and painful tears during the initial writing; and Mocha, who unleashes new and profound feelings of motherhood within me every single day.

And to Kenna, who took a leap of faith in supporting this book right from the start.

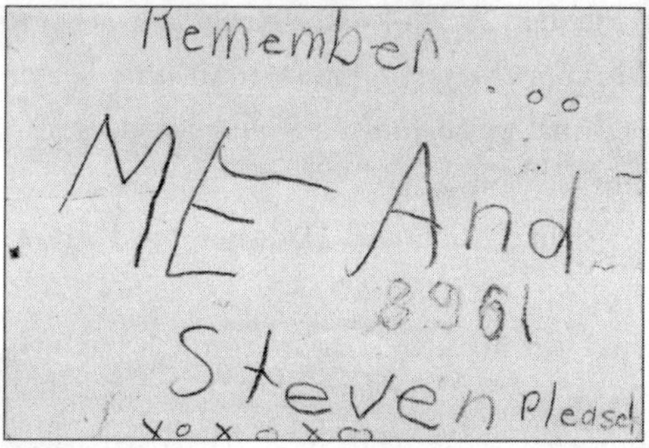
Remember
ME And
Steven Please

Prologue: Against the current

"My mind is troubled like a fountain stirred,
And I myself see not the bottom of it."
[WILLIAM SHAKESPEARE — *Troilus and Cressida*]

[1994] I HAVE LONG grappled with an unnamed entity. It is only now, at the age of 32, that I am gradually beginning to identify what that is: I have never processed the first 20 years of my life and the way they have shaped me as an adult. It was during those two decades that my family was plagued by my mother's recurring bouts of clinical depression. In the years since then, we have very much stagnated in that disease's formidable grip without truly understanding why.

Following a very fine thread, life is rife with symbolism. Writing teaches me to no longer dismiss, but to embrace, significance. On occasion, that significance is felt in the security bars on the basement window that faces out to the ravine behind my Etobicoke house. I look up from my writing desk: the very desk transported from my parents' Hamilton home to mine, and at which as a child I sat and counted my coloured Laurentien pencil crayons — one for each thing Mom was unable to do when she was sick.

My eyes move beyond the beige painted bars to where the clear blue sky dodges the clouds. No matter — the clouds are on a journey elsewhere, and for now, blue sky will prevail. Yet there were times when the clouds did not drift past; they hovered, and smothered all snippets of blue — Mom's favourite colour. How isolating, to harbour not a single shade of sky, day after day ... week after week ... month after month ...

Closed behind the dreary bedroom drapes. Suffocated between the flimsy hospital curtains, which served as poor excuses for privacy from outside stares. Trapped within the horrible headlock of electrodes. Confined to the place nobody talked about. That place where you can still find blackened bars on the windows so the "crazy" people can't get out — for fear they may try and touch the blue sky. What damage did those bars on her mind deliver? What hideous message did they pummel into her head? Wondering how those bars betrayed Mom's sense of sanity and dignity torments me still.

Mere months after my first explosive run at scribbling down memories to form the framework of this book, I began to feel uncomfortable with the disturbing pattern that was emerging. I soon identified the need to turn outward to somehow legitimize my recollections, as if to confirm that things really had been as I remembered them.

One of the first validations I received was in speaking with one of my family's closest friends and a longtime neighbour. On a warm summer evening in June, I summoned the courage to pay her a visit with the express purpose of telling her about this book. As we sat in her living room, a frequent safe haven in my childhood, I nearly dropped the mug of beer she'd offered, when she solemnly remarked, "I wonder how you kids did it." Hearing those words as an adult proved to be the key that unlocked the floodgates of pent-up emotions. I broke down without shame and cried. For someone to acknowledge how difficult it must have been to grow up in a home dominated by depression and its mad sister, chaos, resonated powerfully within me. I knew then I had always longed for someone to voice something to that effect.

Shortly thereafter, I took a bus trip up to visit my paternal uncle and aunt, who live in the Ottawa Valley region. When I revealed to them what I was working on, they assured me, "You have every right to do this; tears have to be cried. It didn't start overnight and it certainly won't end overnight either."

To be sure, the legacy of my mother's depression lives on in these years of her relative wellness. *Afraid of the Day: A Daughter's Journey* is but my own rite of passage toward understanding the insidious and complex nature of that legacy. Where this book began as a catharsis, it soon materialized into a dream that one day, someone would see it in a bookstore, or find it on a library shelf, and know it was written for them.

Part I: To touch the blue sky

One: Eyes of the storm

Waking one Sunday morn in a cold sweat; the eyes of her illness forever seared in my memory . . .

GROWING UP in the shadow of a depressed mother conditioned me to be on the lookout for the telltale signs of her illness recurring. Throughout childhood I would feel like a spy, scanning for clues that Mom was not far from relapse. Before I was old enough to recognize the onset of depression in her pale blue eyes, as I would later become unnervingly skilled at doing, there were indications in the missed appointments and an increasing number of chores left unattended to during the day. By far the most obvious omen was when Mom would stay in bed longer than usual in the morning. She would not be up to participate in the daily routine of making Dad's brown-bag lunch and thermos of black tea; nor would she be lined up with my younger brother, Barry, and me for a dutiful hug and a peck on the cheek, as Dad went off to work. When she was sick, everything suddenly screeched to a halt, like clothes that had jammed in the rollers of a wringer.

When I tentatively entered her room in the morning after Dad left, Mom would ask me to set the buzzer on the kitchen stove, which we commonly used in the absence of an alarm clock. When it shrilly echoed through our ranch-style bungalow, I would listen for sounds of her rousing up while I busied myself preparing for school. As minutes passed with no audible sign of her rising, I pretended perhaps she just didn't hear the makeshift signal, and I would head down the hall to let her know it had sounded.

Not budging, she would ask me to reset it, which I would obediently and repeatedly do, until, with a sinking feeling, I knew she would not be waving to Barry and me from the living-room window that day. We often left for school while she remained curled beneath the covers.

[APRIL 1994] *Passing kids playing after school, I feel emptiness for a time I do not associate with such frivolity. Rather, my 4:00 memories from childhood are clouded with shadows of uncertainty, which loomed over me as I made the dreaded walk home from school. Would Mom be up?*

That question naturally tormented me even more on the days when Mom was still hibernating in bed when Barry and I set out for school in the morning. Dawdling to avoid going home, clinging to the security of a friend's company, sometimes stealing a few extra moments in the sanctuary of their home. How I came to dread the 3:45 p.m. bell of freedom at the end of the school day. The apprehension in the pit of my stomach when I would see the front drapes still drawn as I approached the house. Dragging myself around the back, daring to look up to find her bedroom curtains also closed. Entering that darkened house as still as death, to find the toaster still on the counter, breakfast dishes still in the sink and Mom still in bed. No wonder Barry always took even longer than me to come home.

Slowly hanging up my coat on the hook beside the back door, undoing my shoes, placing them neatly on the rubber mat so as not to leave any mess. Up the two steps into the kitchen and then automatically down the hall to Mom's room. "Hi Mom," I'd whisper toward the bed, where she lay facing the wall as I had left her hours before, as if she hadn't moved at all. As I stood in the doorway, she'd twist her body around to look up and murmur "hi" back.

"Aren't you feeling any better?" I'd foolishly ask, for obviously she wasn't. "No," she'd respond, eyes trying hard to focus on me. "Did you take your pills?" I'd inquire, as if I had every right to do so. Usually, she'd wanly respond that she had, though chances were she had not spoken with her doctor, which followed as my next question.

Beyond that brief exchange neither of us knew what else to say. Before I left her room, stinging tears welling up in my eyes, I'd ask if she needed anything, knowing by heart she'd just want me to start something for supper. I would, of course, glad for a reason to turn away from the haggard, vacant face that gazed back at me. And which scared me. When I could, I would then hurry to tidy up the kitchen before Dad arrived home from work at precisely 4:45 p.m., in an attempt to make it seem like Mom had at least done something during the day. I was not always successful. Sometimes, Dad would arrive and catch me in the act. He was barely in the door before he demanded where Mom was. How I hated to confirm what he too must have wrestled with all the way home.

Thermos slammed on the table; coat shoved into the front closet; footsteps storming down the hall to their bedroom where Mom remained fetal-like. He would start by confronting her in a tone of voice laced with frustration, which gradually escalated in decibel. Not surprisingly, his shouts were to no avail. Those suffering from clinical depression do not respond in favourable fashion to any amount of verbal combat. I could do nothing but desperately try to drown out that horrible, hollow wail as Mom tried to resist Dad's efforts to get her up. "*Let me beeeee!*" she would scream out, often lapsing into a chanting-like rhythm as Dad became more aggressive toward her. Some days, it was worse than others. Lunging toward the bed, Dad would yank her up, pulling her toward the door, forcing her down the hall. Ever so weak and wobbly, Mom would try desperately to press herself against a wall. With her nightgown askew, eyes wild, and hair matted, she would strike out at Dad as he tried to pry her away. At some point during the melee, Barry would have wandered home and I'd motion him to stay with me. Mom would cry out to us both from where we remained frozen in the kitchen. With sickening apprehension, we could only inch toward the hall, pleading with them to stop. Before long, Mom's adrenaline would deflate, and she would revert to her previously withered state, exhausted by the forced exertion.

Eventually, Dad would withdraw, equally spent. He would then resign himself to prepare supper, or take over what I had already started. Monday, Wednesday, Friday were standard fare: bacon and eggs; chili con carne; fish and chips respectively. Other days, it could be leftovers, or whatever was glumly sought out from the freezer. Not that it mattered. From an early age, mealtimes were generally unpleasant. Mom's empty chair and the dismal mood that reigned made it a far from appetite-inducing occasion.

Although Dad was often angry at meals, other times he was intensely sad, pleading with us kids to eat. Despite the discomfort of choking down food past the lump in the throat and into a stomach riddled with knots, we were never allowed to miss a meal. It sometimes took Barry and me forever to force-feed ourselves. Which one of us discovered the nifty little trick of burying the impossible last morsels into our serviettes, I'm not sure. Pretending to have obediently cleared our plates, we would then hide the evidence in the bottom of the garbage can, trying not to think about all the kids in the world Dad frequently reminded us were starving. In retrospect, the stage was set for his daughter's disordered eating patterns, which became full-blown many years later.

Around the dinnertime, I would venture down the hall to offer Mom something to eat. She rarely accepted; usually all she would take throughout the day was a cracker or two to accompany her pills. Periodically, she would come out to the kitchen to fetch the meager ration herself. When she did surface, the tension was palpable; what bitter battery of words would combust between my parents? With any luck, they ignored each other, and while I hoped each time she appeared that she might stay up, I was admittedly awash with relief when she retreated back down the hall to the cocoon of her bed sheets.

More often than not, I had no choice but to take Mom in whatever she wanted, be it an arrowroot or saltine cracker along with a small glass of juice. Torn by the desire to help her yet also afraid of her, I lingered not in that room that oozed sickness and hopelessness. Sensitive to Mom's need for quiet, I would softly ask her if the TV or the music were too loud, offering to close her door before leaving. Sometimes she did not mind if the sounds of another reality drifted in, and I would leave the door slightly ajar, which meant I would have to tiptoe past so she wouldn't hear me going into my bedroom. How I envied Barry the position of his room, because he did not have to pass Mom's in order to reach his; he did not have to resist the urge to glance quickly toward the figure heaped on the bed when the door was left open.

Other than those fleeting interactions, our contact with my mother through the duration of her cycles of depression was limited. The only time we might see Mom again during the course of a day was before bed, when Dad would ask if we had said goodnight to her. I think it was his way of reminding us that we were not to abandon our mother.

Regrettably, sometimes I could only bring myself to call in to her darkened bedroom from the hallway between our rooms. Wary of her by day, I was afraid to go near her by night. Seldom were there the hugs offered she so desperately craved. How that must have hurt her terribly.

What she needed most from my Dad, my brother, and me was for us to be there for her: to sit with her and hold her hand, to reassure her of our love and our presence. But we unwittingly isolated her within the confines of those four cream-coloured walls; trapped by our fear of an illness we didn't understand.

Such is how the days would pass, governed by this pattern that could last for weeks on end, until Mom was either hospitalized, or the shock treatments she received on an outpatient basis finally kicked in. Before such relative calm prevailed, we would all be ripped through an emotional hell I would wish upon no one. Each of my parents fought so desperately, with such misdirected energy, to surmount the impossible. They simply had no idea how to cope with my mom's repeated cycles of virtual incapacitation. Sadly, our household was lacking some of the fundamental ingredients conducive to a successful healing environment for those suffering from severe clinical depression: patience and compassion.

When depressed people perceive that those closest may not care about them, it intensifies how despondent they already feel about themselves. Unwittingly, our family dynamics fostered that sense of reality in Mom. On some level, she must have been aware of her young children's fear and ambivalence toward her. There was certainly no mistaking or escaping her husband's combustible temper, as the profound helplessness and frustration of having a chronically ill wife was often released as explosive fits of rage.

The yelling penetrates the seemingly cardboard-thin walls of my bedroom. Finally, I can stand it no more. I creep into the hallway, terrified of what I will see in the living room. Mom is hunched in the corner of the couch, flailing up at my Dad as he tries to pull her up to get her to do something — anything. I can only stand there trembling, sobbing, "Please stop, please don't," fearing one or both of them will be injured, leaving Barry and me to deal with the aftermath . . .

*[*ESTER SUNDAY, LATE 1960S*] Sitting cross-legged on the living-room floor, doing my best to assemble my newest acquisition: the miniature pieces of yellow plastic doll furniture spread before me on the coffee table. Vainly trying to shut out Mom and Dad fighting in the kitchen. Unable to take it anymore, I flee to my room, tears streaming down my face. How could the Easter Bunny bring such bittersweet gifts?*

Looking back, the frequency with which such verbal and physical altercations arose was alarming. Even now, as those and other scenarios reappear in my mind, I must tightly blink them into obscurity. Much as I may have wanted to, and as some kids actually do, I was afraid to run away. With the exception of the neighborhood Terryberry Library, where I would sometimes take refuge, there was nowhere to escape for any significant duration. Fortunately, those were the days when a young girl could walk unaccompanied to and from the local library, even if it was a good 20 minutes away. Once there, I could hide myself away between the shelves, where an intangible comfort settled over me. How I loved that place. I decided that if not a teacher, then I would definitely become a librarian when I grew up.

Nonetheless, seeking solace in the security of books was also a lonely and time-limited experience. Sooner or later, the library closed for the night and it was time to return home. Though the walls were never thick enough, I spent most of the time in my bedroom. Beneath the makeshift tent I would create, or in the back of my closet where I kept a little stool, the tears would flow. And I would wish it all away.

Two: Shock after shock

Eight o'clock hospital hand — and they still have not come back to visit me ...

OFTEN AS I may have sought the solitary refuge of my bedroom or the library, where I could be alone with my fear and sadness, early on, I harboured an inordinate dread of being left alone.

A routine childhood operation in December 1967 proved to be a cornerstone in my five-year-old life. My parents had taken me to the Hamilton General Hospital one afternoon in preparation for a tonsillectomy the following morning, promising to return after supper to visit. How vividly I remember the agonizing wait for them to reappear in the ward playroom. While all the other kids were glued to the television, my eyes were riveted to the oversize clock on the wall above. As the hour hand reached 8:00 my heart sank: visiting hours were over and they still had not come. I was inconsolable as the nurses tried to assure me that my parents would soon arrive. The weight of anticipation and ensuing anxiety proved too much for my young self to bear. I was sobbing uncontrollably when Mom and Dad finally arrived moments later.

Such an excessive outburst can only be attributed to an internalized fear of abandonment, the seeds of which had been planted at birth. As Mom struggled through a depressed state of being, triggered by my 1962 emergence from her womb, it was as if her subsequent physical and emotional distance from her newborn robbed us both of the precious opportunity to fully foster the essential postpartum bond.

32

She was hospitalized three months after my birth on March 17.

From infancy, it was as if I acquired an acute awareness of her absences, whether to bed for days or weeks, or to the psychiatric ward of various Hamilton hospitals. As I grew older, I would also worry about her ultimate departure: death. In one cruel, and at the time, not so unusual way, Mom had already started to sneak off. Over a 20-year period, she endured hundreds of shock treatments; after each one, a little bit more of her fizzled away.

In December 1962, Mom was subjected to her first round of electroconvulsive therapy (ECT), at the Hamilton Psychiatric Hospital. One of the few flashbacks that surfaces for her most readily of that first ordeal, is that of an 80-year-old woman, restrained upon one of the gurneys lined up in the dingy hallway. Mom remembers being surprised for some reason that someone that old would be given shock treatments. As Mom bided time until her number was called, no amount of mental preparation could have possibly alleviated the blind anticipation of her initiation into the world of shock. With alarming clarity, Mom recalls nervously telling the doctor who hovered in angelic white above her "I'm still with it you know," anxiously awaiting the anesthetic that never came. Instead, what followed were explosions of every colour, in an attempt to shatter the fragility that engulfed her new motherhood.

... a needle plunges into a thread-like vein, bleeding muscle relaxant into her body ... thin hands neatly folded over her sunken stomach fail to smother the rumbling hunger pains ... she's not eaten for hours ... chalky aftertaste of the sedative as it sticks to her parched mouth ... melancholy eyes staring up in fear of the unknown ... a tight-lipped nurse to her right in a seriously starched white dress rubs cool jelly-like cream on each temple — to hasten the current and prevent the burn ... the grim-faced reaper on her left reaches for the headgear shaped like a huge wishbone, and lowers it into position, one electrode on either side of her forehead where the jelly marks the spot ... a rubber gag placed in her mouth so the tongue will not be

swallowed . . . or bitten off . . . the eyes of those above her meet and blink their accord . . . oblivious to her muted pleas to wait . . . she's still awake . . . with the flick of a switch on a gleaming metal box, the electricity peels through her brain . . . two seconds in time that last an eternity . . . her body surrenders to crudely choreographed spasms . . . fists clench and arms curl repeatedly up and down her torso . . . head rolls from side to side, eyes screaming in shocked white silence . . . the damage done . . . the rubber removed . . . the danger averted . . . her mouth left gaping, loosely opens and closes in a vain attempt to speak from the comatose state that sets in . . . the minutes tick by . . . she awakens to be wheeled out to the hall where she'll sleep for another two hours . . . and she'll remember nothing of this terror — at least so they say . . .

How old were we before we knew where Mom was going every Tuesday and Friday morning for weeks at a time, maybe once or twice a year? How could we have known that as we played at recess with friends, she lay alone, shackled down to a hospital bed as volts of electricity ripped through her brain?

When Barry and I were well within our first decade of life, all we knew was that on those mornings, Dad took Mom over to the Henderson Hospital because she was sick. Hustling his wife out of bed and out of the house all before 6:45 a.m., he would return some 30 minutes later to get his kids ready for school before he went to work. By the time we returned from school in the afternoon, Mom would have come back by taxi. But she was not always "better" if the series of treatments had just started. Usually, she was back in bed and with a splitting headache to boot.

When my brother and I were older, we learned the reason for these headaches was the bilateral shock treatments she received in the hopes of eventually burning through her debilitating bouts of depression. Sometimes, weeks would pass before she was finally back to what we deemed as "normal." But how can normalcy ever be regained when the brain is repeatedly eroded with electricity — surely more than the delicate tissue was ever intended to withstand? To paraphrase Ernest

Hemingway, who succumbed to the electrical storm of 11 shock treatments before his death several days after the final currents were administered, the cure may be brilliant, but the person is lost. To this day, Mom is adamant that she would never wish ECT upon anybody.

I'll never forget one of the first indications that Mom's brain was damaged. Still in our pre-teen years, Barry and I were sitting with Mom at the dining-room table when somehow the conversation turned to a digital clock radio. With a puzzled look on her face, Mom innocently asked Barry what "digital" meant. How could she not remember what such an everyday object was? Barry laughed and thought she was joking; something told me she wasn't. In hindsight, though we may not have thought of it as brain damage, it definitely registered with both of us that something was not right with Mom's brain.

Over the years, time and again, there were similar clues that betrayed that portions of Mom's knowledge base had been wiped out. Still, almost without exception, when the depression would not lift for weeks on end, ECT was ultimately reverted to as the treatment of choice by her psychiatrist of the day. In turn, our family became mired in a love/hate relationship with shock therapy. Much as we may have hated or denied what damage ECT did to her mind, what the bi-weekly shocks eventually did for her depression was paramount. Sooner or later she was "better" — at least until the next time. But the bitter reality of a repeatedly electroshocked mother is that my brother and I would never know her any other way. She had left before we had a chance. In our youthful minds, we knew her only as a mother unlike any other.

I am called down to the principal's office. My brother Barry won't stop crying: he wants to go home. His kindergarten teacher, Mrs. Yoshida, is trying to contact Mom. There is no answer. Do I know where she is? I mumble something of a response, knowing I will have to take him home myself. Clutching his small hand, running across the park as fast as our little legs will take us, for I must make it back before the final 9:00 a.m. bell. On the way home, we pass my classmate Todd, who asks me where I am doing. I choke out a response, asking him to please tell Mrs. Bacon, our second grade teacher, that I won't be late; I just have to take my brother home. The burning tears of shame for doing what a mother is supposed to, blind me.

Like an albatross twisted around my neck, I carried that desperate need to simultaneously cover up, yet deal with, what was happening in our family: in retrospect, a tall order for a short, shy little girl. But the weight of responsibility became my self-accorded cross to bear.

When people called and Mom was sick, how I hated to have to tell them, almost apologetically, that she was not well. It was understood what *that* meant. Cancelling appointments with her hairdresser, dentist, and doctor was equally discomforting: how I wished the world did not have to know that Mom was "not feeling well" again. Although people were not aware of the exact nature of her illness, they knew something was wrong with Mrs. Bonner.

At Buchanan Park, the public school my brother and I attended in the 1960s and early '70s, there was a real sense of community. There were plenty of "stay-at-home-moms" who were involved in many of the school activities: chaperoning on class trips; supervising the lunch room; working at Saturday afternoon matinees in the gymnasium; baking for different occasions; coming out to attend play-day at the end of the school year. It filled me with equal portions of shame and sadness that everybody else's mother except mine was able to participate. Similarly, I remember bursting with pride on the rare occasion when she was like a regular Mom, such as the day she took her turn to watch over the kids in the lunchroom. That token appearance meant the world to me. But those instances were sadly few and far between, not only for my brother and me, but also for Mom. If her lack of participation made us feel different from the other kids, it most surely distanced Mom from her neighbourhood peers, and eroded her sense of belonging in the world around her.

For all intents and purposes, during Mom's years of depression, we were an island unto ourselves; the severity of our family situation was kept closeted at all costs. Neither Dr. Robert MacIntosh, our long-time family physician, nor any one of Mom's string of psychiatrists over the years, ever saw fit to bring us together to talk about depression, our fears and struggles to cope with it and with life in general. We were increasingly enmeshed in the web of an insidious illness we couldn't comprehend, let alone explain to others. Some well-meaning friends and family — even doctors — referred to Mom's depression as "another one of her spells"; an ironic choice of words, for it was as if a spell had indeed been cast upon her and she underwent a total transformation. She was not our mother, but a woman whose presence became all too familiar...

Three: Under lock and key

... they have imprisoned her, and changed the rules of her life ...

ON MARCH 24, 1930, Martha Bonner was the first of two children born to Elsie and Albert in east-end Hamilton. Photos taken during the late 1950s depict my Mom as a radiant young woman: fresh-faced with a toothy, almost impish grin. Her clothes were well tailored and her hair neatly curled in the style of the day. Before she was introduced to my Dad, Mom had never really dated much. Rather, her life revolved around her job, family, and friends. She led a rather sheltered life; her identity was somewhat overshadowed by her more outgoing younger sister, Iris. Nevertheless, her friends paint a picture of my Mom as the unassuming life of the party, who loved to go out to the movies, bowling, and (much to my dismay), wrestling matches! One friend laughs as she recalls how much Mom enjoyed sitting ringside, cheering on her favourite wrestler.

On the other side of town, Henry Reid was born April 12, 1930, to Robina and Jack. Henry and his younger brother, Russell, were well liked in their west-Hamilton neighbourhood and among church members and schoolmates. Kick the can, hide and seek, bicycle riding, and ice skating in Victoria Park are among Henry's fond childhood memories. In contrast, an unsmiling Sea Scout stares back from the brownish-tinged photos of his youth. Beneath the surface, Henry carried the weight of an unhappy home life upon his stocky young shoulders.

Henry was introduced to Martha on a blind date in 1957. On the surface, they seemed to have things in common. Both were 27 and born under the sign of Aries. Neither had completed high school — not unusual in the post-war 1940s — but had entered the work-force at the age of 16 to help support their respective families. Mom worked in accounts receivable at Hamilton Hydro in the downtown core, and Dad was a draftsman at Bridge & Tank in the northeast end of the city. With his sense of humour and generosity, Dad quickly won my Mom's heart. For better, for worse, in sickness and in health, they were married at Zion United Church after barely a year of courtship.

Their May 3, 1958, wedding photos portray a beaming young couple eager to begin a life of their own. Though it was the company policy of Hydro for married women to resign, Mom was able to find a comparable position at Slater Steel, where she worked until leaving to start a family. By the fall of 1960, Martha and Henry were settled on the west Hamilton mountain in a neighbourhood that would later become known as Buchanan Park. Their ranch-style bungalow was one of the first houses to be built in that area during the 1960 upheaval of apple orchards and farmers' fields. By all accounts, they were a happy pair, and would often spend time with two or three other young couples who have remained their lifelong friends. Early photos of their first few years together capture a playfulness that would never be fully regained. For after I was born, March 17, 1962, something went awry. Their St. Patrick's Day baby did not bestow upon them the luck of the Irish.

She cradles her not with a mother's loving arms, but gazes upon her with disdain ...

My parents brought me home from Hamilton's Henderson Hospital on March 24, 1962; one week to the day since I'd emerged from the womb. It was Mom's 32nd birthday. Her mother, Elsie, came up to give her eldest daughter a hand with the newborn, whom they named Nancy. During the first week of my homecoming, I developed a severe case of infant colic. This alarmed my parents, and they summoned Dr. MacIntosh, their family practitioner, to the house. The cause of the colic was difficult to pinpoint and there was no absolute cure. My parents were simply forced to endure what is commonly deemed one of the most difficult infant syndromes. The stress level between them was acute, and, like most colicky newborns, I perhaps sensed the household tension and cried even more.

Looking back at photos of Mom in the weeks following my birth, there is a hollow happiness etched in her face. She looks down at me placed in her lap, or beside her on the couch, as if uncertain that I am truly hers — wondering what on earth she has done. She does not cuddle me with maternal warmth and a joyful smile, but tentatively props me up with a rigid hand and a mournful gaze. An excessive worrier by nature, Mom fretted over whether, as two novices, she and Dad could properly care for a newborn. Her anxiety intensified to the point where she would not let Dad leave the house, convinced something would happen to me if he were not there.

Charged with a colic-ridden baby, whose incessant wailing was as merciless as nails raked down a chalkboard, I cannot help but wonder whether she meant misfortune at the end of her own hand.

For several days in succession, Henry pacified Martha by staying home from work and keeping watch over their infant daughter — and her mother.

Mom's fragile state was further tested by the death of her maternal Grandmother on March 27, 1962. Mom had been extremely close to my Great-Grandmother, whom she fondly referred to as "Nan." Emotionally, psychologically, and physically, Mom's plate was overflowing during my first month of life.

Through the spring, as my mother became increasingly overwhelmed and unable to cope with what was happening within and around her, she began taking to her bed for days. After several weeks of this pattern, hospitalization was eventually deemed the only recourse. In June 1962, Mom was first admitted to the psychiatric wing of the Hamilton General Hospital. At a time when she should have been in the prime of her life, she was caught in the merciless grip of a faceless villain who would shadow her for years to come. It was conceived as I was, and accompanied me into the world, transforming the lives of my parents almost overnight. From the embryonic stage of uncertainty, through the fetal phase of anticipation, the burden gestating within my Mom had been only briefly guised by the miracle of childbirth. It was not long before the flame of joy diminished and the veil of hope disintegrated, exposing an alien in their midst. It is unfathomable how bewildering that time was for them. Suddenly, they were not just new parents; they were a worried and frightened young couple who knew not what the next 20 years would entail.

Though an estimated 50 to 75 percent of new mothers experience sadness and unstable emotions in the days following childbirth, within a couple of weeks, the blues have passed, as the hormones revert to their pre-natal state. However, for some 10 to 20 percent of postpartum mothers, the emotional turmoil, which typically sets in at some point during the first six months, endures. Unlike the more common postpartum blues, postpartum depression can become progressively worse as it gives rise to disturbed sleeping and eating patterns, evokes feelings of worthlessness, interferes with the new mother's ability to think clearly, and riddles her with anxiety about motherhood. In some cases, the mother is so severely depressed she may be unable to care for her baby. If such a depression is not accurately diagnosed and properly treated, it can linger for months or even years. My mother's would linger for years.

With his wife hospitalized, Dad was faced with the dilemma of what to do with Nancy. When he could, he kept me at home with him. It was a strain, however, because he was working all kinds of overtime to earn extra money. Dad credits his boss' understanding with keeping him from "going bats," as he struggled to balance everything between home, work, the hospital, and me, wherever I happened to be. I was moved around a fair bit, mainly between Mom's parents' in Hamilton and her sister Iris' family in Grimsby, some 20 miles away. Though Iris and her husband, Ron, were themselves parents of a year-old infant, Chad, she and Mom were close, and would do anything for each other, not the least of which was taking care of each other's children.

As the summer of '62 unfolded, there were no proud mother outings in the warm sunshine. Instead, the baby stroller remained tucked away, in anticipation of the day Mom might join in the sidewalk chats with the other young mothers in the neighbourhood. She suffered a heavy blow to her pride in having others take care of her newborn while bearing the shame of being held hostage on a psychiatric ward. In July, there was yet more upheaval in Mom's life, when her father, Albert, suddenly passed away at the age of 60. In a strongly medicated state, Mom was released to attend the funeral. At the gathering afterwards, Dad recalls Mom being so "stoned" that she paid no heed to his warnings and gulped down two bottles of beer before being taken back to the hospital where she stayed for the remainder of the summer. Unable to properly grieve her father's death or to lend support to her own mother compounded the postpartum depression. It was as if the seeds of happiness my parents had worked so hard to sow were crudely dug up before they had a chance to securely root. After Mom was released in August, both my parents had appointments with Dr. MacIntosh at least once a week. Yet despite that frequent contact, there was never any concrete explanation for what was happening to my Mom.

In December 1962, Mom was again hospitalized. This time, it was to the Ontario Psychiatric Hospital, barely a ten-minute drive from my parents' home. She was assigned a patient number, and the home she shared with my Dad was referred to in government correspondence as "her former address." Family and friends were confused. What was wrong with Martha? One of my mother's high school chums, Marjorie, was incredulous at Mom's second hospitalization; this certainly did not sound like the carefree woman with whom she had vacationed in Bermuda five years ago. In stark contrast to that holiday of lounging upon warm tropical sands beneath clear blue skies, my mother spent her baby's first Christmas and New Year locked away in the "crazy house."

Mere days after Christmas, Dad was notified that, due to his wife's admission to an Ontario psychiatric institution, and in accordance with The Mental Hospitals Act of 1960, the Public Trustee had assumed custody of Mom's estate. Dad was, therefore, duly obliged to complete the requisite government questionnaires and provide detailed information pertaining to her financial affairs. In early January 1963, Dad received a phone call from their bank manager, who had the regrettable task of informing his client and friend that my parents' assets were frozen. The bank had been contacted regarding Mom's institutionalization, and was required to remit all balances, securities, and safety deposit box holdings to the Public Trustee, as well as statements reflecting all transactions on Mom's accounts over the previous three-month period. No money was to be drawn or cheques written on accounts, joint or otherwise, bearing Mom's name. Faced with the seizure of funds reserved for mortgage payments and other household utilities, Dad wrote to the Public Trustee, with the hope that the decision would be reconsidered. He fully expected, since Mom had been allowed some weekend passes home from the hospital, that there had simply been an oversight.

On February 15, 1963, Mom was granted probationary discharge to Dad's care, at which time he again sought to have the money in their account released. As he had heard nothing from the Public Trustee, Dad then contacted his member of provincial parliament, who agreed to pursue the matter on my parents' behalf. On February 25, 1963, the issue was raised on the floor of the provincial legislature. While the actions of the Public Trustee were in place to protect people incapable of taking care of their own affairs, the MPP pleaded for common sense to be adhered to, in an instance where there was clearly a family member capable of handling such matters. Furthermore, their MPP questioned why the bank had to be directly involved, as it would have been far better public relations for the Trustee to confer directly with the clients themselves. It would also have spared his constituents the humiliation of having such a private affair made public to the bank through the grapevine of tellers. In summary, the member for Hamilton-Wentworth cited government lack of insight and wisdom for causing undue hardship to a family that was already under enormous stress and strain.

The Attorney General, under whose jurisdiction the Public Trustee was legislated, conceded that, of the 18,000 patients who were at that time wards of the Public Trustee, some cases did warrant closer scrutiny. In so doing, there were those, such as my Mom's, whose files could have been granted more compassionate consideration. The House agreed that in the future, better communication was in order between the bureaucracy responsible for administering the particular sections of the Mental Hospitals Act, and those directly affected by it.

Nevertheless, as Mom's probationary period did not expire until August 15, 1963, the funds remained frozen until such time as she was completely discharged and the Public Trustee ceased to have control over her affairs. When activity had not resumed to their joint account by the beginning of September, Dad wrote directly to the Attorney General, documenting the steps he had taken since the previous December. A response acknowledging Dad's letter was followed by a second one dated October 16, 1963, in which it was confirmed that funds had since been deposited back into my parents' account. The Attorney General thanked Dad for bringing the matter to his attention and in the same breath, hoped that my father could appreciate the vast amount of paper work involved with a file of this nature, which had contributed to less than prompt action. To add insult to injury, there was no interest paid on the money during the time it was seized, and a compensation fee was outstanding to the Public Trustee for supposedly acting on Mom's behalf. Furthermore, my Dad was outraged to find typing errors in the numerous pieces of government correspondence involved in the ten-month process.

As their first 18 months of parenthood foreshadowed, depression would not be an incidental happening in the world of Martha and Henry; it would grow to monumental proportion, organizing their life, tangling them in an ever-taut web of disarray. Even the infant in their lives was affected by the upheaval, exhibiting signs of extreme shyness well before the age of two. Nellie Burgess, a long-time family friend, recounts how I would hide in the back corner of the car whenever my Dad took me anywhere. On the occasions we visited her home, when Dad was finally able to coax me out of the Ford, I would reluctantly emerge from his car to their couch, where I stayed curled up like a dog until it was time to leave; a puppy prematurely separated from a mother unable to engage her in the maternal weaning process.

Four: A playmate for Nancy

[DECEMBER 1964] *Clinging to the back of Grandma Bonner, I peer expectantly around her, waiting for the front door to open. They're here: Mom and Dad stand proudly in the vestibule, my brother a babe-in-arms between them ...*

DESPITE THE harrowing episodes of depression following my birth, my parents decided to have another child. One friend of theirs recalls telling Dad she thought it was absurd for Mom to risk another pregnancy after what she had endured the first time. When I asked Mom many years later whether or not she had been apprehensive about having another child, she replied no. They'd wanted a little playmate for me. However, Mom did confess to family members at the time that she hoped her second pregnancy would not be the same. Whatever apprehension may have been harboured was alleviated by Dr. MacIntosh, who assured them that everything would be fine. Two years and nine months after I was born, my brother Barry came into the world, December 10, 1964. As fate would govern, the arrival of my brother gave birth to yet another bout of depression, thus leaving another unweaned puppy to fend for itself.

While my parents struggled to cope with the unpredictable nature of Mom's illness, there was enormous pressure on Dad. By the time my brother was born, the roller coaster ride of despair had taken over his world. Yet when friends and family asked after Mom, many fearing the worst, Dad refused to accept that Mom was on the verge of another setback.

When Barry and I were young, Dad's brother, Russell, and his wife, Barbara, offered to take care of us while Mom was sick and to give Dad a break. Dad would hear nothing of it, his pride preventing him from accepting the support he must surely have needed. It was a vicious circle, perpetuated by the need to have control over his responsibilities and the fear of losing it. Over the years, the only people Dad really ever relinquished his care of us to for any duration were our Grandmothers. During the week, one of them would come up and stay with us if Mom was in the hospital. On weekends or school holidays, we would go down to stay with them; but it was only at Grandma Bonner's we would stay overnight. There we would be free to play and eat our favourite foods, stay up late and forget about why we were there.

Much as I loved my Grandma Reid's home with the large front verandah and massive chestnut trees, the inside seemed dark and mysterious. The heavily draped windows shut out the light in a way that reminded me of home when Mom was sick. Ironically, though I was so fascinated with her eclectic possessions and Scottish ways and even grew to be very much like her, I was afraid to spend the night — something that must have hurt her deeply. But in her old country wisdom, I believe she understood that no harm was intended, as everyone tried to make the best of a bad situation.

Other times, Dad might take us to spend the weekend with our Aunt Iris and Uncle Ron, and our cousins Chad and Dale, to their wonderfully huge new home in Burlington. Barry and I always looked forward to those times, though the pretense for being there was often a sad one. How I envied my cousins, with their rooms full of the newest clothes and toys, and parents who didn't seem to argue. But as with the journeys to Grandma Bonner, all good things had to come to an end and it was back to the house on the hill.

Five: Wolf in sheep's clothing

"Dirty rotten kids!" Mom is seated in a corner of the kitchen, looking like a wild
animal as she spews out those blood-curdling words for no apparent reason. I cry, "Be
quiet, be quiet," ashamed that my cousin Chad is here to witness this side of his only
aunt. Running downstairs to comfort my brother, Barry, who has fled to the
basement, desperately trying to explain that Mom doesn't really mean it — in spite
of the fact I am afraid she does . . .

[SUMMER 1994] Writing beneath the cherry tree in the backyard, my
stomach seizes as the peacefulness of the early June morning is broken
by the sound of the woman's raised voice, slamming doors, and a car
speeding off. The shock of hearing that outburst was that it was a
mother yelling at her kids; there is something far more disturbing to
me about a mother's raised voice than a father's.

When Mom was well, she never seemed to really get mad at us.
With the exception of washing Barry's mouth out with soap for
swearing (something she nevertheless found difficult to do), Mom
never yelled, spanked, or punished us. I cannot recall ever arguing with
her: she always seemed so fragile. Yet when Mom was sick, it was as
if all the little pills she ingested joined forces, conspiring to over-
throw her normally complacent personality. Medications that ran the
gamut from antidepressants to tranquilizers to antipsychotics.
Tofranil. Elavil. Norpramin. Nardil. Trilafon. Librium. Thorazine.
Haldol. Each in their turn, these and other tiny soldiers on the
kitchen counter, rose to the challenge of combatting the relentless foe

of depression. As was common with many of the antidepressants at the time, she tolerated side effects including dry mouth, diarrhea, and dizziness. During one of her hospitalizations, she had such a violent reaction to the antipsychotic drug Haldol, she almost bit off her tongue. Were it not for the frantic shouts of a fellow patient that summoned a nurse in the nick of time, she may have succeeded.

Another time, Mom, Barry, and I were visiting Grandma Bonner. We were in the living room watching TV when suddenly, Mom started to make odd, gagging noises. Turning toward her, we watched in horror as her face contorted and lockjaw set in. In a panic, we called Dr. MacIntosh. Arriving at Grandma's later that evening to assess the situation, he gave Mom a muscle relaxant and struck yet another medication from her "Okay" list.

The twists and turns in Mom's face that day symbolized everything we were afraid of: that she was not really who she seemed; that at any moment she would change again and be lost to us forever. I cringe to think how ill-informed my parents were about the potential side effects of her medicine. In retrospect, the promiscuity with which the doctors prescribed her medication was no less than appalling. There was every indication that Mom was frequently overmedicated, particularly during periods when she would barely eat. In bed for days on end, often the only nourishment she would take would be a cracker or two and some juice. The less she ate, the more weight she lost; the less she weighed, the more concentrated the drugs in her system. The more heavily medicated she became, the more her personality altered, as aspects of her we did not normally see surfaced. She did and said things uncharacteristic of her. Repeatedly, she'd lapse into a pummelling of her thighs or banging the side of her thin body against the wall in expressions of sheer despair. The self-inflicted bruises betrayed a mental torment we did not understand. The shaking and shrill voice, which came out of her, was not really our Mom. Depression swallowed the person we knew and loved.

Much as I was uncomfortable to admit it, that unpredictable side of Mom gave me reason to fear her. When she was sick, I was afraid to do anything that might draw out the demonic-like side of her. And yet, the painful occasions did present themselves when I had to betray her. Although she wanted nothing more than to be left alone in her bed, there were times when I could no longer stand passively aside as she sank deeper and deeper into the depression. From the lone telephone on the kitchen counter, I would stretch the cord as far as I could. Crouched behind the china cabinet, I made every effort to muffle the grinding of the plastic dial. Excruciatingly slow, I dialed those seven numbers to the outside world, usually a desperate call to one of her doctors. Despite attempts to conceal my act of treason, Mom's hearing seemed to sharpen. She would first yell from the bedroom for me to hang up, then weakly make her way down the hallway, pleading me to stop. Between sobs, I would try to convince her to speak with the doctor. At times, I felt she must have hated me, as my guilty eyes met hers, which blazed with hostility.

Broad daylight. Doing the dishes. Shamefully on my guard. Ears perked up for the sound of footsteps in the hallway. Eyes furtively glancing from the soap-filled sink to the reflection in the window ahead of me. Heart pumping when Mom comes into the kitchen behind me. I spin around to face her, dish soap dripping on the floor, certain the fear in my eyes registers in hers . . .

The unforeseen and irrational anger born of the depression evoked a disturbing distrust in Mom. I felt particularly uneasy whenever my back was turned. Through the night, when especially vulnerable, I would desperately try to convince myself I was imagining things. No matter how tightly I squeezed my eyes shut, the visions of Mom coming in my room wielding a knife prevailed — an omnipresent dread that cloaked me like a second skin.

[MARCH 1996] A chilling déjà vu resurrected that childhood phobia. A neighbourhood woman in her early thirties, in the midst of her own battle with manic depression, spent a couple of hours sleeping on my living room couch one stormy spring afternoon. Knowing she was not well, I let her sleep as I carried on with the dishes. All the while, I was acutely aware of how my ears were cocked to the sound of her rousing so I would not be taken off guard. I chided myself for allowing the past to taunt me like that. But it did. I was not immersed in the dishes as much as in my own recurring nightmare of the past; I failed to hear her as she crept into kitchen behind me. I froze at the sound of her voice. Heart racing, I whipped around in a state of panic, a fistful of cutlery and an expression of guilt to greet her: thank goodness I had already washed and dried the large cutting knives. "I'm sorry, did I startle you?" she asked sleepily, her eyes roaming my kitchen for evidence of something she might be able to eat. Red-faced, I assured her she had not, hurriedly relieving myself of the potentially lethal weapons. Overreacting though I knew I was, I could do nothing to turn off my imagination. Offering her the banana she had spied and another cup of tea, we went back into the living room, and sat down facing each other.

Growing up, however, there was nothing a cup of tea could ever hope to quell, neither the fear of Mom hurting us, nor the fear for her own safety. When she was sick, she would announce things like, "If I don't get up tomorrow, may I be struck dead" and "You'll be better off without me." Fearful of what she might do, I tried my best to reassure her that she was needed and loved. But she was beyond reason; there was no consoling her when she was trapped in that blackened crevice of negativity.

One Christmas, Dad, Barry, and I came home from visiting the Caldwells, our family friends, to find a kitchen knife with a scorched tip on the counter. With visions of the worst in our heads, we raced into Mom's room. Another false alarm. We found her as we had left her several hours before, huddled beneath the covers. When asked what had happened to the knife, she was unable to explain exactly why she had stuck the instrument into the hallway socket. But the hideous reality could not be dismissed. Whatever her motive had been, she could have electrocuted herself. For some inexplicable reason, that same knife remained in the drawer for years afterward, until it was finally discarded. How many times my hand passed over it, pushing it aside in search of another, a grim reminder of what could have been. How often I dared to think that maybe it would be for the better. At least the torment would be over — for all of us. By some twist of fate, she held on; more often than not, thanks to the relative safety of a hospital psychiatric ward.

Six: Behind the painted line

"Remember . . . Me and Barry Please! xoxoxo"

WHILE PUTTING together a family album one Christmas, I came across a creased photo of Barry and me, he in his crib and I standing beside it, holding on to the side rail. On the back, those few words and the year 1966 were printed in thick letters penciled by my four-year-old hand. I'd wanted Mom to keep it while she was in the hospital, just so she would not forget us.

The shame of Mom's illness and fear of her hostility and self-destruction were replaced by profound loneliness and sadness every time we entered the sterile environment of the Henderson Hospital. The all-too-familiar drive along Concession Street, circling the block until a free parking spot could be found. Through the revolving door, we solemnly paraded down the main corridor, past the gift shop, and toward the elevator that would all too soon grind to a halt at the fourth floor. With stomachs twisting and hearts aching, the three of us stepped off into

Ward 492: the psychiatric ward. With the familiar smells of mental decay assaulting our senses, we slowly made our way down to Mom's room to drop off our coats.

As hospital rules prohibited patients from staying in bed during certain hours, we usually found her sitting and waiting in the sunroom at the end of the hall. We would awkwardly greet her, conscious of the stares from the forgotten souls not quite so fortunate to have visitors. Each time, we made sure to take her something: a package of Kerr's licorice allsorts; Planter's peanuts; a current issue of *People Magazine*, an unsqueezed tube of Crest toothpaste; clean clothes; a handful of dimes for the phone. Mom has never been a reader at the best of times, so books and crossword puzzles were out of the question. She was not one for repetitive and time-consuming activities such as knitting or crocheting. Neither did she engage in the common psychiatric behaviour of chain smoking to while away the infinite hours passing time still considered as living. So aside from the essentials, what else can you give someone who is so often in the hospital? At the beginning of each stay, we would bring her a carefully chosen cactus garden. From its place on her bedside cabinet, the brightly painted figurines perched upon the coloured gravel would watch over her, keeping her company when we could not.

If Mom had just arrived, those initial visits were terribly strained. Dad, Barry, and I were all still battle-weary, from whatever chaos had precipitated her admission, but at least the situation was now out of our hands. We made small talk. What she had for dinner. What we had for dinner. What we did at school. Who had called. Dad's curling games. The weather. Sometimes she would show us a hospital craft she was working on. I will never forget the leather wallets with the embossed flower patterns, and the day she proudly presented them to us: a black one for Barry and a tan one for me. When we were at a loss for things to say, fortunately, there was always the TV to grab our listless attention and sometimes spark a few sentences.

On the days when she received her shock treatment, our visits were cut short, for she needed more sleep than usual afterwards to nurse her splitting headache. Much as I ached for Mom to be back home with us, sometimes I was thankful for the excuse to leave her where someone else could take care of her. Furthermore, visiting Mom was confusing and frightening. Barry and I were aware of the other patients watching us. Although taught never to stare at strangers, sometimes we couldn't help but sneak a peek at them. Those who gazed with empty eyes through their own reflection in the window out into the dead of night; others who chain-smoked without noticeably blinking or breathing; some who obsessively paced up and down the hallway; those who scrutinized us as we feigned family closeness. It was hard to comprehend how Mom was like all these other inmates scattered around her: she always seemed to be the most "normal" person there. It must have been doubly alienating to be separated from her family, and to be shut in with people so unlike her on the surface: alcoholics and junkies; paranoid schizophrenics and manic-depressives; those with scarred wrists — some newly bandaged. Something about seeing Mom in that "safe" environment was horribly cruel: she just didn't belong.

Nonetheless, Mom always befriended people when she was there. By nature, she is a caring and kind-hearted woman, the type that people just naturally speak to at bus stops or in grocery lines. As I got older, I found that other patients would adopt Mom as a mother-figure or confidante. Among the many world-weary souls whose lives crossed hers, I recall two women in particular: Connie and Mavis.

Connie was in and out of the hospital over the years for depression, just like Mom. On more than one occasion, they ended up in at the same time, and I began to look for her familiar face when visiting Mom. She spoke often of her violent marriage, which I know was unsettling for Mom. The last time I saw Connie, I was in my teens. She lay bruised and bandaged in the bed diagonally opposite from Mom's. Time passed and I remarked that Mom never mentioned Connie anymore. She'd died. Mom had not wanted to tell me. Her husband had finally made sure she'd never see the inside of hospital walls again.

My memory of Mavis is of a very poor and lonely woman. Like Connie, she grew quite attached to Mom during their mutual hospitalizations. Having no children of her own, she took an almost grandmotherly interest in hearing about Barry and me. When both were out of the hospital, Mom visited her at home when she could, and once I asked to go along with her. Mavis lived alone in a rather unkempt apartment in a sordid area of downtown Hamilton. The day we called in, I was shocked to see her body grossly bloated from water retention brought on by a bowel obstruction. I couldn't wait to get out of there, yet politeness and pangs of sympathy hampered my escape. On the way home, I told Mom I'd like to give Mavis two cushions I had recently made in home economics class. But her death was imminent, and I never had the chance.

Knowing Mavis and Connie, I dared to think how much better off Mom was than both of them — two women whose lives were wrought with misfortune. As sick as Mom was, she seemed to have so much more going for her than either of them.

As Mom became stronger throughout the course of each hospital stay, her true colours flourished in striking contrast to the tattered souls around her. But that time could take weeks, composed of our numerous visits. In an innocent attempt to salvage the situation, it dawned on me in the sixth grade that I could get away with wearing blue jeans to school when Mom was hospitalized. That was something not allowed when she was well, for she always made sure that Barry and I were dressed neat and tidy; blue jeans didn't classify as such.

But I would have forsaken the forbidden Lee jeans with the smooth thick leather patch on the back waistband forever to have Mom better and back home with us; never again to leave her on the other side of the thickly painted line on the speckled tile of the hospital floor, which warned against her freedom, crudely marking the place just beyond the phone booth where she would line up with other patients, waiting her turn to make precious calls home. Heart-breaking moments ensued as we hugged her one last time, and waved to her until the crushing instant when the elevator doors clanged mercilessly shut.

Seven: Shame of sickness

"Get up!" "Do something!" "Snap out of it!" "Shake it off!"
Words yelled at Mom as if she were a dog . . .

IT IS A disturbing commentary on the medical profession of the 1960s, '70s, and even into the '80s, that those very words were uttered by the likes of both family doctors and psychiatrists toward a person suffering from major clinical depression. Depression was not regarded as the widespread and debilitating illness it is today. Rather, people suffering from depression, my mother included, were often made to feel as though the illness was their fault. My mom was seen as a weak woman who simply lacked the will power to get out of bed and get going. Frequently, she would lament, "nobody understands." She was right. For many, a severely depressed person's reality, and meaning of the word "can't" is beyond comprehension, even to those who are trained to know better.

At some point in their lives, most people will experience the feeling of being down in the dumps. Between 5 and 10 percent of the population will succumb to the black and bottomless hell of depression. There are few illnesses of its magnitude: a place where there is no sun; hopelessness prevails; self-esteem is paralyzed and suicide beckons as the only viable means of escape.

Although family and friends are frequently in a position to provide some degree of support and assistance, they often don't know where to start. They may offer advice that they genuinely believe will help the depressed loved one feel better: "maybe if you got up and washed your face"; "perhaps try getting dressed"; "how about going for a walk?"; "why not take up a hobby?"; "just think on the bright side." For those in the depths of depression, there is no bright side. When well-meaning friends and family find their words ring hollow, they may turn away in helpless frustration, depriving the sufferer of critical human interaction.

I cringe to think of how tormenting it must have been for Mom to have nobody understand or even believe the gravity of her illness. Especially the doctors. She was relegated to an isolating and lonely existence by the very professionals deemed licensed to help her. Despite all the years of pills, shock treatments, and hospitalizations, it was as if her doctors were merely grasping at straws each time another episode occurred. For all intents and purposes, depression was trivialized as a female problem, little understood by a profession largely dominated by insensitive males who were no more than pill-pushers and zappers. They didn't even have the sense to provide either of my parents with resources to help them learn more about depression and family functioning.

Although four lives revolved around whether or not Mom was sick, depression was largely considered to be only her problem. It was dealt with in a vacuum that virtually ignored how the other family members may have been affected. The one brief exception to this was a visit to Dr. Newt Simpson, the psychiatrist Mom had for many years, whom I would later dub the "Candy Man," for the way he doled out shock treatments as if they were indeed candy. If we had met Dr. Simpson with any preconceived notion of learning more about Mom's sickness by means of our day-to-day experience of living with it, we were woefully misguided, for that meeting served only to establish a negative stereotype of psychiatrists it would take years for me to break. I can still picture the diminutive man with the plaid pants, checked jacket, and mismatched tie, speaking to us across a desk cluttered with files.

That Mom's life was somewhere on that desk was hardly reassuring. We left his office with little hope there would ever be an end to the nightmare. If anything, his approach to Mom's illness demonstrated a blatant void of insight and compassion into the harrowing effects of depression on the woman we loved, and on our family as a dismembered unit.

Surrounded by doctors who didn't seem to be genuinely concerned about Mom's harmful cycles of illness, our family was virtually left up the proverbial creek without a paddle; navigating waters made murky by insecurity, uncertainty, and shame. Over the years, my brother and I could only huddle helplessly in the trenches, witnessing our parents desperately wage a war they were ill-prepared to fight. And we kept it all to ourselves.

In retrospect, that shame and sickness went hand in hand was not restricted to Mom's depression; it was an association I made with respect to myself as far back as elementary school. Most kids love being off school sick, because it entitles them to watch TV for hours on end, eat only their favourite foods, thus garnering the envy of schoolmates. To the contrary, I hated to miss school, for it set me apart from my classmates in a way I was not comfortable with: sickness meant you were different. Just like Mom was different than other moms when she was sick, I too felt alienated from my friends when I was ill, and I cowered under the attention it drew to me.

[KINDERGARTEN, 1967] *Lining up in front of our teacher, Mrs. Yoshida, so she can make sure we are all properly bundled up against the bitter December day before heading home for lunch. As my turn comes up for inspection, she innocently announces that the raspy voice I have acquired after my tonsillectomy makes me sound like a little boy. I cringe as the others around me giggle ...*

[GRADE 1, 1968] *During a phys. ed class, I jump off the stage and twist my ankle. I'm taken to the nurse's office, then home, where I have to stay for a couple of weeks.*

One day, my teacher, Mrs. Mockler, comes over with my homework. When I see her coming up the front porch from my vantage point on the couch, I make a mad dash into the kitchen, defying the pain in my foot, lest she see me in my pyjamas: the ultimate shame, of course . . .

[GRADE 3, 1970] *When I catch the chicken pox just before Christmas, life at school goes on without me, even the* Mary Poppins *play in which I was to take the role of the mother. My classmates write me letters, telling me about the play, and that they have learned to borrow in arithmetic. They and Mrs. Studinski, our teacher, hope I'll be better soon. I am heartbroken to be missing all the fun . . .*

In each of those instances, being sick isolated me. It was not a matter of other kids making fun of me, for I was well liked. Rather, it was how my perceptions so easily became my reality: that there was shame to be felt in being sick.

The shame of sickness was heightened when Mom was in the hospital. Never latch-key kids, we would often be taken in after school by our Great Auntie Annie, who lived over on the other side of the park, on nearby West 5th Street. A wisp-like, wizened little woman who smoked the old Vantage cigarettes with the circular filter in the end, she would entertain us with stories while we waited for Dad to pick us up on his way home from work. As fond as I was of her, I wished I didn't have to explain to our friends why we were going home the wrong way. I felt like it was written all over my face that our Mom was too sick to take care of us. Even years later in high school, getting off the bus two stops earlier than usual to transfer to another, my friend Wendy asked me where I was going. I was too ashamed to tell her I was going to visit my Mom in the hospital.

Any shame about the nature of Mom's illness was reinforced by the commonplace jokes kids would naively make about the "O.H." — the Ontario (Psychiatric) Hospital. Though kids will be kids, and even many adults are not above insensitive remarks about psychiatric hospitals and the people in them, I always made a conscious effort to refrain from making such comments. Unbeknownst to them, those jokes were far from funny to me, for they cut into a hollow and vulnerable spot deep within. It was a terrible secret that my Mom had been in the O.H., or any other hospital psychiatric ward. I believe this struggle with shame underlines how alone we all were in trying to cope with the stress of Mom being sick and the stigma of mental illness.

As far as I knew, we were the only family going through this ordeal. With one exception.

When I was in Grade 7 or 8, I learned that the father of my classmate Kate was on the same hospital ward as Mom. In a warped, selfish kind of way, that was reassuring for me: there was someone else with a parent like Mom. Although Kate was not in my immediate circle of friends, I regret that I never spoke to her about it. God knows it would have alleviated some of the tremendous shame and isolation I felt. Maybe I could even have helped her when she most needed it a few years later.

How much precious energy could have been saved had we understood the nature of the beast that stalked my mother, and shadowed us all. In our ignorance, we did all the wrong things. Life was lived walking on shards of glass, never knowing what tomorrow would bring.

Eight: Between a hope and a prayer

[SUMMER 1969] *In Mom's darkened bedroom, a man I barely know somehow entices her to come out among the living after days upon days in bed. It is a miracle that he is able to do what neither the drugs nor her doctors have succeeded in doing of late . . .*

THE SAVING grace over the years was those friends and relatives who weathered the storms with us. Those like Mrs. Burgess, who brought over casseroles to console us while Mom was in the hospital. And the "mystery couple" who arrived on our doorstep from half a world away to pray for Mom. The miracle worker was in fact was my Dad's uncle Alex. He was a Presbyterian minister, visiting from Australia with his wife, Belle, my Grandmother Reid's sister. They had stopped over in Hamilton for a visit with my Grandmother and upon hearing of Mom's illness, had asked permission to come up and speak with her. When the minister emerged from Mom's room, he announced to those of us waiting anxiously in the living room that she would be out shortly. To our utter amazement, several minutes later, out Mom came to wash herself, staying up long enough for us to have wondered what on earth this man from a land down under had said to her. Whatever was shared will remain forever a mystery. Had the word been in my vocabulary at the time, I would have called it an exorcism, albeit a temporary one, as the next day, Mom once again took to her bed.

With that one exception, I never associated Mom's cycles of wellness with anything religious. Beyond that brief encounter, I was disillusioned with religion. Granted, I may have periodically thumbed through the cream-coloured Bible, complete with golden-trimmed pages, real pictures and a zippered close that was kept on the dining room bookshelf. I even diligently tried to follow the daily reading schedule in the pocket size *New Testament* the class was given in fourth grade, and would kneel down to say my prayers each night, long after Dad stopped reminding us to do so.

Yet the professed virtues of prayer were inconclusive as far as I could tell; after all, Mom was never better for very long before another one of her spells came on. Hence, organized religion never played a significant role insofar as providing the guidance or solace we so desperately needed. Rather, I learned very early to associate religion and church with frustration and sadness. It was in a back pew of St. Andrew's Church, which we attended for a brief time in the late 1960s, that I saw Dad praying with tears sliding down his face. I had never before seen him cry; I assumed he was silently pleading his case for Mom.

Our own prayers seemingly unanswered, it could be said that we depended upon others for that spiritual strength. The Hodgesons were one such couple. Despite the significant size of their own family, Mr. and Mrs. Hodgeson, our "surrogate grandparents," had unlimited capacity to bring others into their fold. During our pre-teen years, spring break visits to their home in Flint, Michigan, brought welcome reprieves from the isolation that our family dynamics tended to foster. They seemed to be the only people who had equal compassion toward both my parents. Although they had known Dad first many years ago in Hamilton, they betrayed no favouritism. When Mom married Dad, she too became part of their extended family. Once inside their home, a comfort unmatched surrounded us. Gangly Mr. Hodgeson, with his grandfatherly smile and soft-spoken words of wisdom, liked nothing more than to draw pensively on his Camel cigarettes while doing crosswords, or playing pool with Dad, Barry, and me. Rotund Mrs.

Hodgeson, with a perpetual gleam in her eye, would cook up a storm while she chatted with Mom about everything from African violets to recipes for her trademark dishes and bargain hunting at Meijer's. Barry and I loved to sit up on the high kitchen stools, where we could listen for hours as Mrs. Hodgeson's hearty laughter soothed the heaviness that perpetually lingered beneath our skin.

Despite their open invitation to stay with them, we usually bunked at the nearby Farm Motel. On the one occasion that we did accept the offer and spent the few days at their home, Mom took to bed. It was difficult for everyone, but the Hodgesons provided a buffer effect, easing the usual tension between my parents when Mom was sick. Mrs. Hodgeson was very protective of Mom, and gingerly took her under her wing until it was time to leave. Despite the cloud that hung heavily over that trip, the Hodgesons always loved to have us visit them. I think it used to break their hearts when it was time to release us back into the vast emotional trenches of Ontario at the end of our visits one week later. Many tears were cried all around when we said our goodbyes each year in their driveway.

At one point in the early '70s, Dad drove down to the Hodgesons by himself to have some time alone. I wrote a letter to Mrs. Hodgeson, thanking her for giving Dad a place to go. She responded that they were simply affording Dad time to rest and do whatever he chose, not letting him talk much so he could concentrate on something other than the situation at home. "We feel truly sorry for your Mom too. We can't understand why this has to be, only God knows. We wish it could be different and we know you and Barry must be suffering too. May God in his wisdom help you all. We will pray to that end," she wrote to me on her trademark flowery notepaper, which I have kept to this day.

Despite the distance that separated our families, we maintained strong ties with the Hodgesons until their deaths in the late 1980s. When they each passed away, it was as if a huge part of our small family died with them. Our relative agnosticism aside, we had always derived profound support and comfort from them; they were truly angels in our midst.

Closer to home, our earthly strength was derived from a street full of wonderful neighbours. Although many of them were on the outside looking in, a select few knew more of what was going on behind our heavily draped windows than others could only guess. Contrary to a host of doctors who dealt with Mom and dismissed our worries, time after time, open doors and outstretched arms of neighbours consoled us when the heart could bear no more, or the kids had to be sheltered.

Hurriedly making our way with Dad down the street. Arriving at Mr. and Mrs. Thames' front door, Dad's tears betraying an urgency they immediately understand. They usher us inside and Mr. Thames leads a frightened Barry and me up into the living room, offering us something soothing to drink. In the background, Dad's troubled voice barely rising and falling as he speaks to Mrs. Thames. Then he is gone. Barry and I curl up on their window seat, where we wait and wait until it is safe to go back home.

Not only have the Thames and my parents taken care of each other's homes during vacations for the better part of 40 years, but Evelyn and her late husband, Bob, also consistently offered a strong support mechanism for our family. They were particularly helpful for Dad when Mom was not well. So that Barry and I were never left alone, we would often go there while Dad went to pick up one of our grandmas to look after us while Mom was sick, or if he had to take her unexpectedly to the hospital, probably yanking her up out of bed, forcing her to get dressed, then pulling her kicking and screaming out to the car. Whether or not an ambulance ever came to cart her off in her agitated state, thereby relieving Dad of the dirty deed, I have never had the courage to find out.

In the calm of the Thames' warm and comforting blue living room, Barry and I would wait until Dad came back. At other times, their house provided the refuge Dad so often needed — somewhere he could go to vent his fears and frustrations, leaving Barry and me back at home with Mom. I think that Mr. and Mrs. Thames probably knew more about our family than most of our friends and neighbours.

From time to time, Mrs. Thames would come over to stay with Mom while Dad was at work and we were at school, just in case she needed anything. Never one to impose on others, Mom would always say, "If you don't mind, I don't really feel like talking." She was always apologetic, Mrs. Thames remembers. "That's okay, I'll just read the paper," she'd gently reassure Mom. And that she would do, particularly on the days when Mom came home after her shock treatment with a pounding headache and feeling totally disassociated with the world. "Those treatments tormented her," Mrs. Thames recalls. Although she didn't understand anymore than anyone else about the nature of Mom's gruelling depressions, her compassion was a sustaining force in our lives. Decades later, when I expressed long overdue gratitude to her for looking out for us as she did, it was she who had sombrely remarked, "I always wondered how you kids did it."

Perhaps we "did it" because we didn't know any differently; Mom's depression could surface at any time of year. Some, like Mrs. Karsson, our next-door neighbour, remember the patterns of Mom's illness were like clockwork: every spring and fall. "She could never have worked," she once ventured to me, "the depressions were too frequent. It must have taken a toll on your Dad, with pressure at work and also having to take care of you kids." If it was taking its toll, we all tried damned hard to hide it.

[AUGUST 1994] *I find myself engaged in the mundane chore of sewing buttons on a favourite top long held together by a pin or two. With the exception of ironing, sewing anything is the domestic chore to which I have an innate aversion. Yet that morning, I was distinctly aware of how relaxed I was, tending to the truant buttons while silently musing, "You can't mend clothes unless your mind is mended." My thoughts drifted to a recent conversation with Renée Karsson, a neighbour of my parents, and how she had always associated mending with Mom's level of wellness.*

For more than 30 years, Mrs. Karsson has watched our family grow, struggle, and drift, acquiring a sixth sense in the process about what was happening behind our four walls of brick. Over the fence, she and Mom would share the trials and tribulations of motherhood. Periodically she would invite Mom over to share a beer in the heat of a summer afternoon. More often than not, Mom would decline, saying she had some darning to do. Although Mrs. Karsson would encourage her to bring it along, Mom always seemed to have other things to do that kept her inside. When Mom was slipping, Mrs. Karsson could always tell by her eyes, in the way the pupils became like pinheads and her gaze was dark and vacant. It became all the more apparent that darning was a refuge more than a reason. As a child, I remember Mom sitting for hours on the chesterfield, black and white wicker sewing basket at her side, surrounded by heaps of socks that begged her attention. When she was sick, even mending the darned socks demanded more than she was able to give.

As I learned more about Mom in those early days of my childhood, a picture emerged of a timid young woman who wanted desperately to be a good mother and housewife. My Aunt Barbara remembers how obsessive Mom was about cleaning. Both she and my Uncle Russell tried to convince Mom she was expecting a lot of herself with two young kids on the go. They contend that Mom never had a sense of her potential as an individual outside the marriage, and that the constant cleaning, laundry, ironing, and the like were what boosted her self-esteem. When she was well, Mom operated on the notion that you never knew when someone might come over, so the house always had to be tidy. And tidy it was. When my brother and I were young, Dad would often photograph us sitting on the living room coffee table in our "Sunday best." Mom kept the table so well polished that you could see our reflections staring up at us in many of the photos.

Tending to the house was also a way to please my Dad, whom many thought of as a very harsh, quick to temper, controlling man. I cannot help but wonder whether Mom was afraid of him. Although certain relatives and friends would tell Mom she shouldn't let her husband talk to her the way he habitually did, for Mom to be anything less than submissive was out of character — and out of the question for many housewives of her generation. Pressuring herself as she did with housework only complicated matters, because she felt she could never do enough. When that self-defeating mindset takes hold, it is crippling, and can trigger periods of depression in those inclined toward introversion. When depression loomed for Mom, the anxiety would intensify, as she felt herself lose control over the very things she depended on for her sense of self: tending to the needs of her children, her husband, and the house. The wheels were set in motion for the depression to take over: the less she was able to do, the less she did and the more vulnerable she would be to the downward swings. It was a dizzying spiral that was eventually all consuming and people around her could only watch helplessly.

Nine: Naming the nightmare

From the darkened living room, I listen to Mom in the lighted kitchen, calling people with almost an urgency, to let them know that "they" have finally given her a name for "it": chemical imbalance in the brain . . .

AFTER SO MANY years tortured by an unnamed entity, how relieved Mom was to find out that what she experienced in the form of debilitating depressions was indeed a bona fide illness. How that day finally came be, I cannot be sure. What I will forever remember is the vignette of me on the other side of the kitchen wall, hearing Mom call friends and family, one after the other, to share with them in a voice peppered with unmistakable relief, the news of what was wrong with her. I too was relieved, because the depressions had become insidious recurring nightmares for our whole family. I was most happy for Mom; this was long-awaited proof that she really couldn't help herself. It was as if she was finally being vindicated for all those years of people telling her to "snap out of it" and "get moving." At long last there was something concrete to offer as an explanation for her "spells." Given that we had the fancy-sounding reason for her depression, I think there was an assumption that Mom would magically get better. No more days and weeks in bed, no more hospitals, no side effects from drugs that didn't work, and certainly no more shock treatments. The doctors would now be able to fix Mom.

Unfortunately, naming the nightmare did not expedite the miracle cure we so naively anticipated. As it turned out, nothing much changed. The depressions kept coming. There was no definitive drug to help her. The hospitalizations continued. And it took more and more shock treatments to obliterate each cycle of depression.

Furthermore, in their infinite ignorance, the doctors still did not see fit to take measures to help our family understand the intricacies of this newly defined cause. If anything, learning about the chemical imbalance only raised more questions. Was it something the body brought upon itself? Could it be triggered by people? Certainly many blamed Dad for his demanding ways, and the frequent verbal assaults he hurled towards her. However Dad's treatment of Mom may have influenced her depression, all we were told was that there were some foods, such as chocolate, that Mom was now not allowed to eat. Other foods, such as tomatoes and chicken, were only to be consumed once every five days, as if different foods were responsible for bringing on the mysterious imbalance. Even to this day, the occasional person will innocently ask if we ever found out whether the chocolate caused Mom's depression. We remained very much in the dark about what this "chemical imbalance in the brain" really meant insofar as why depression reared its ugly head at regular intervals.

Depression is most readily associated with its recognizable signs and symptoms, such as disturbed sleeping, eating, and thinking patterns, and also isolation and apathy. The causes of depression, however, are often addressed as the secondary focus. At one time, depression was classified as either "exogenous" or "endogenous." Perhaps the most familiar form of depression is exogenous, whereby depression manifests itself as a reaction to an identifiable external stress, or significant loss, such as death, divorce, or unemployment. Conversely, as was the case with Mom, endogenous depression is caused by a chemical imbalance in the brain. Endogenous depression can be an inherited illness, in that there is a genetic predisposition to altered brain chemistry. Chemicals called *neurotransmitters*, such as serotonin, are at insufficient levels in the brain and affect the production of positive feelings. Peacefulness, happiness, and hope are replaced by despair, fear, and worthlessness. These days, it is no longer easy to differentiate between kinds of depression, because the illness is regarded as a combination of factors biological, psychological, emotional, and situational in nature. Although depression is now one of the most readily treatable maladies, Mom would continue to be taken over by the depression for years to come, before a "cure" would be found. We continued to live in reactive mode, moving through the world governed by its crippling cycles.

Ten: Not enough coloured pencils

"God grant me the serenity to accept the things I cannot change, the courage to change the things I can, and the wisdom to know the difference ..."

SUCH WAS inscribed the plaque with the praying hands given to Mom by Mrs. Karsson; the "Serenity Prayer" as it is widely recognized. For many years, it rested quietly on Mom's dresser, silently beseeching us to accept that her depression was something beyond her ability to control. Much as I tried to embrace the philosophy, I was no less vulnerable to the desperate pangs of wishing she were like other moms. But those years were wrought with unfulfilled wishes.

Sitting at the desk in my bedroom, counting the new pencil crayons I had received in my Christmas stocking. I finger each of the smooth, slender Laurentien pencils gingerly, carefully setting one aside for each of the things Mom can't do when she is sick: one for cooking; one for dusting; one for cleaning the bathroom; one for vacuuming; one for laundry; one for ironing; one for dishes; one for grocery shopping. As my list grows, I eventually run out of colours.

My heart sinks. Dad comes in my room and I hastily cover up what I am doing in overwhelming guilt, as if he can read my mind ...

That guilt was a heavy cross to bear. I was ashamed of myself for even daring to tally all the motherly things Mom was not able to do. Yet I could not deny the difference between my Mom and my friends' moms: that innocent act of counting pencil crayons made it all the more concrete. And yet, when Mom was sick, she never really asked

Barry and me to do anything specific: we just instinctively knew what was expected. Roughly translated, it meant pitching in to help Dad with all the chores represented by those slender pencils, in addition to the obvious tasks of making our beds and keeping our rooms tidy. On hot summer days, it meant maintaining stifling silences, tiptoeing through the house and not throwing rubber balls against the back wall. We kept our friends outside: they wouldn't understand, for neither could we.

[JULY 1994] *During a therapy session with a counsellor named Claire Richardson, I was encouraged to talk about the good things I remembered that Mom used to do. I was taken aback. My silence shamed and embarrassed me, for my memory of anything potentially positive was tarnished by her illness. I panicked: surely there must be something. I scanned the past like a public library microfilm, searching for the elusive. Tears welled up and threatened to wash away what fragile snippets were flailing their way to the surface. Strangely, many recollections revolved around food: those chewy Quaker Oats ready-mix oatmeal cookies she'd make by the dozen; the perfectly layered chocolate dominoes that occasionally nestled on the bottom shelf of the fridge in anticipation of Christmas company that seldom came; the thin-crusted Chef Boyardee pizza suffocated with tomato sauce and onions; Kraft macaroni and cheese; take-out Chinese and the other "forbidden foods" Mom, Barry, and I would indulge in when Dad wasn't home.*

The next several frames consisted of the little things Mom has always had a particular knack for buying: stocking stuffers, birthday cards, and mementos for every occasion. I vaguely remembered bus trips to the Rockton and Caledonia fall fairs, summer excursions to the CNE, and tickets to see one of her favourite performers, Burton Cummings. But those shreds of hazy memories occurred only when she was able to get up out of bed and participate in the life around her. They are mirrored images of a mother trying so damned hard to please others that her effort was still palpable, as I sat facing Claire with tears rolling down my 32-year-old cheeks. Though jaded be my recall, anecdotes from friends and relatives help shed light on the more pleasant times so long overshadowed.

In between Mom's episodes of depression, she and Mrs. Karsson have had many laughs over the years. Mrs. Karsson recalls the "girls' nights out" when some of the neighbourhood women would go to a movie, out for dinner, and, on one (?) occasion, they rallied their nerve to see the infamous stripper "Mr. T" at a pub not far away.

My childhood friend Elaine also associates Mom with food, claiming she made the best lunches. After her mother returned to work, she and her younger brother Brian would sometimes come over when Mom was able to fill in for their regular lunch sitter. Along with Barry and me, the four of us would spend the lunch hour listening to Partridge Family albums and watching the *Flintstones* — after we'd eaten of course. The standard fare at our house during those "festive" lunches with Elaine and Brian would include Pizza Spins, Bugles, Bits & Bites, grilled cheese sandwiches, french fries, and, best of all, Mom's homemade pound cake, which Elaine loved to coat with mustard. Now a dietitian with a notorious passion for junk food, Elaine laughingly claims she was initiated into the world of fast-food indulgences at my house! Although I do recall those lunchtime escapades for four, I cannot help but wonder how difficult it must have been at times for Mom to fulfill this commitment to Elaine's mother when she could feel herself slipping.

Over the years, there were Mom's brief forays into a number of hobbies that were barometers of her wellness. In the mid-seventies, Mom joined a women's softball league at nearby Buchanan Park. I was so proud of her, as in my close circle of girlfriends, only my friend Lori's mother ever took up the call to bat. No matter that Mom was relegated to right field or that she was not a very strong or confident player; at least she had the courage to try, swinging the bat as if her life depended on it. In a way, perhaps it did. For the season or two she played, she was a part of something. But a baseball cap cannot for long shield the wearer from the blues bubbling inside.

Curling was also something Mom briefly dallied with, though more at the urging of Dad than a compelling desire to learn. I have no doubt that the curling club experience did not constitute a good time for Mom, for there was an elitism that swept its way across the ice, easily intimidating those who didn't quite fit in. And Mom didn't. She was the wife who was so frequently sick that Dad attended many of the social events without her. Understandably, while the curling club was often a haven for Dad, it was more of a never-never-again land for Mom. I could hardly blame her, for I too sensed the false airs of superiority that gushed among certain members on the occasions I went along to watch one or both parents curl.

I would venture that almost as gruelling as curling were the sewing lessons. Time and again, Mom would pick up sewing projects where she had left off when the depression set in. I think it must have been quite difficult to keep up the pace of my friends Sharon and Elaine's mothers, who were experienced sewers, while she remained a veritable beginner. I will never forget the day she finally finished the full-length, sleeveless, emerald green dress with the sequined trim. It seemed to take her forever, but the day she wore it to a curling club banquet, I was as proud of her in that polyester dress as I was of her in the baseball cap. For I sensed to what lengths she pushed herself, enduring self-induced pressure that she might one day find her niche.

Sadly, the numerous abandoned hobbies would ultimately attest to her losing battle with the recurring adversary of depression.

And so as my life whizzed before me in response to Claire's gentle prodding, I caught glimpses of Mom biding time as the walls of depression rose and her self-esteem crumbled. On the verge of taking to her room, she would pass endless hours on the chesterfield, picking and chewing her nails to the bloody quick, an ominous indicator that depression was yet again clawing its way to the surface.

Eleven: All I want for Christmas

We stand silently at the edge of the driveway, huddled together against the late May chill, awaiting the grand finale, wishing the emptiness could burn away as quickly as the little red school house . . .

ASIDE FROM THE perennial Victoria Day fireworks, Dad always went beyond his best to give us what he could: Valentine chocolates and Easter egg hunts; backyard sandboxes and skating rinks; baseball gloves and swimming lessons; Hallowe'en costumes and back-to-school clothes; birthday gifts and Christmas stockings — we were always well-provided for. Grateful though Barry and I were, it seemed somehow disloyal to enjoy those things without Mom. Especially Christmas.

It is unfathomable for some to imagine Christmas as anything but a festive time of year, marked by traditional family gatherings and good cheer. Yet holiday times are by far the worst for people with depression — and those around them. The mournful melodies synonymous with the spirit of the season serve only to intensify waves of despondency. As Christmas approached, it was indeed more melancholia than merriment for our family, never certain of what the big day would bring.

[NOVEMBER 1994] Innocently catching CHCH-TV news clips of the Santa Clause Parade in Hamilton. I feel the tears slip down my cheeks, flooded with flashbacks of standing in the bitter cold outside

Clines' dress shop, near the north-east corner of Main Street and Kenilworth Avenue in east-end Hamilton. Barry and I would be bundled up from head to toe: warm woollen hats and long thick scarves; Grandma Reid's hand-knit mittens; snowsuits zipped tight until they pinched our chins pink; big-buckle brown galoshes worn over our patent-leather shoes. There we would wait, pressed together with the throngs of other bodies, in anticipation of the grand finale. As a family of four, it was fun to make the trip down to that part of town where Grandma Bonner lived. As a trio, without Mom, it was often a long, cold, miserable few hours, until that first glimpse of the jolly old man whom we hoped would make our Christmas wish come true; a wish that more often than not melted as sure as the first November snowflakes upon the sidewalk.

In the weeks leading up to Christmas, another annual outing would be the excursion down to Robinson's department store, where we dutifully had our pictures taken with the resident Santa. Some years, we must have been whisked in and out for that sole purpose; we are still garbed in winter outerwear, standing or sitting stiffly beside the overstuffed fellow. Otherwise, we were clothed in our favourite outfits, one picked out by Dad, if Mom had taken an early leave of absence for the holidays. Looking back on the photos, I wonder what was going through the minds of my brother and I as we posed stiffly with that magical provider of childhood dreams, our faces stricken with some inner anxiety, somehow doubtful this roly-poly man could really bring what we most wanted — and seldom was it the toy of the year.

[Christmas Eve] Barry and I glued mere feet away from the tv, eagerly awaiting reports of "unidentified flying objects." After firm assurances by newscasters that Santa Claus had indeed been sighted heading towards the Hamilton mountain we faithfully left a plate of Dad's meticulously carved shortbread and a glass of snow-white 2 percent milk on the counter. Permitted to sleep in the same room on that special night, Barry and I tumbled to bed whispering ourselves into slumber, visions of a healthy Mom dancing through my head.

[CHRISTMAS MORN] The first tentative sign that just maybe Santa had granted our wishes was to find the Christmas stockings weighing heavily on the bedroom doorknobs. Eagerly, we two pyjama-clad kids would spill out the contents of the green felt stockings with our names written in glittery silver across the top. Cross-legged upon the bed, we would share and compare our treasures, right down to the large, polished Red Delicious apple firmly nestled in the toe of each sock.

Next, we would tiptoe out into the living room, to feast our eyes upon packages of all shapes and sizes neatly placed beneath the artificial tree of green. Despite whatever fears might have been hovering in the back of our minds, nothing could quite diminish that early morning thrill of Christmas. We would then wait patiently, for Dad — and hopefully Mom — to join us, making just enough noise so there would be no mistaking we were up and ready.

[DECEMBER 1994] Last-minute Christmas shopping. Passing through the accessories department of The Bay, I notice an older man and younger girl, whom I automatically assume to be a father and daughter, trying to decide on the appropriate gift for their wife and mother. In the second it takes for the pair to register in my mind, I am thrown back into the days of accompanying Dad down to Robinson's in Hamilton to find something for Mom. Even when she was sick, there was always something under the tree for her from Dad and us, especially her favourites: Avon bubble bath; Laura Secord assorted chocolates; a bottle of Chablis wine.

With any luck, Mom would be able to get up for the morning ritual of opening presents. So far so good. As she and Dad encouraged Barry and me to open ours first, we could not conceal our joy in between sideways glances over to Mom, where she sat quietly in the corner of the couch. When the floor was sufficiently strewn with crumpled paper and bows, Barry and I then set about arranging everyone's things under the tree. For some reason, it never took long to assemble Dad's: we always had a hard time figuring out what to buy him. If we were really stumped, we sometimes wrapped up one of his hardcover *Reader's Digest*s or a volume of his *Churchill Memoirs*, just to make it look like more. While Barry and I hovered around the tree and Dad prepared the stuffing, the naked turkey remained plumped expectantly on the counter for Mom to begin the salt-water wash. The air was strained as we agonized over whether Mom would be able to stay up, or be drawn back to bed, unable to carry on her role as Mrs. Claus anymore that day.

The bubble burst as soon as Mom announced she was going to lie down for a few minutes. No matter how much we dared to hope, there was no denying the fate of the day. Barry and I stiffened as Dad uttered some frustrated profanity. Abandoning the stuffing, the raging tug-of-war to keep Mom up was sparked. When the rope finally snapped, Mom lay slumped back in bed, leaving Dad haggard and teary alongside Barry and me, the presents mocking us from under the tree; for all we ever really wanted for Christmas was for Mom to be better.

Suddenly, the long-awaited Christmas day could not end soon enough. The twinkling decorative outside lights falsely betrayed the appearance that we were enjoying Christmas like all the other neighbours. Inside, with carols mournfully drifting from the radio through the house — "Silent Night" the worst — we somehow went through the motions of the day, passing restless hours until it was time to go with Dad to pick up Grandma Reid and Grandma Bonner. Christmas dinner was a subdued affair, with Mom burrowed under the covers down the hall. No amount of coaxing from even her own mother, Grandma Bonner, would bring her out to join us. All she wanted was to be left alone, and not put a damper on our day: as if keeping out of our sight put her out of our minds. Nothing could be further from the truth: we were conscious of nothing else.

Over the holidays, there would be the inevitable invitations to visit friends and relatives. Too young to stay home by ourselves, Barry and I glumly accompanied Dad. I felt I betrayed Mom by going, yet even when I was old enough, I was afraid to stay in the house alone with her. During those visits, we were the family with the missing appendage. Everybody knew why Mom was not there, but it was only spoken about in hushed tones so us kids wouldn't hear. I felt sorry for Dad. Although he must have craved the outside distraction of others, whenever I looked at him across a room full of people, there were years of sadness etched on his face. There was nothing to be jolly about as far as he was concerned. The onset of the Christmas season still conjures up a host of heavy-hearted memories. It is as if that first Christmas Mom spent in hospital after I was born in 1962 foreshadowed the pattern for years to come.

Twelve: Beaches of Sauble

[AUGUST 1994] *Lakeside morning jog. I look down into the murky water where I'm able to distinguish ripples of sand beneath the surface, evoking memories of Sauble Beach and the way the water shimmered with the early morning sunshine, flocks of dancing seagulls overhead . . .*

THE ONLY times I really remember Dad's face a little less weathered was during the first two weeks in August. Although there was never any guarantee of Mom's wellness, that period was faithfully reserved for our vacation at Sauble Beach, on the south-west shore of Lake Huron. Before the days of mandatory seat belts, Barry and I used to take turns laying across the cases of Charlie's-brand soda pop, piled two-high on each side of the hump on the back-seat floor during the three hour journey. In my Gravol-induced stupor, I always preferred that spot, because my parents' often-bickering voices from the front were more easily muffled. Finally, the long-awaited red *Welcome to Sauble Beach* sign that spanned the main drag would come into view, the glistening waters of the lake beckoning beyond.

Of the three cottages we rented over some 15 years, the one that fronted the beach was my favourite. It was a cosy, four-room haven, nestled between two sand dunes. Barry and I shared one room, each of us vying for the top bunk. Waking in the morning, the vantage point offered from up top was the ideal barometer of the day ahead. Peering out over the rafters, between towels flung over them to dry, out the window to the lake, we could tell in a flash whether the waves would be in our favour. Calm, sunny days were not surprisingly relished. If I had landed the toss for the top bunk, I'd scurry down the ladder, squirm into my pre-Speedo-era suit, and scamper out to join Dad for an early morning dip. Being early risers, there was seldom anyone else in sight. After a few sturdy strokes and some underwater exploration, it was back to the cottage to rouse up Mom and Barry for breakfast.

For the most part, those holidays were carefree times and the days were never long enough for all we wanted to accomplish. We loved it there: waves and walks; sandcastles and suntans; horseshoes and lawn darts; go karts and harness races; drive-ins and bingo; Saugeen Indian ice cream at Little Beaver's Emporium and flaming roasted marsh-mallows over the bonfire outside the cottage. Even come rainy days, we were not to be daunted. With no TV to indulge us, we spent hours amusing ourselves with books, jigsaw puzzles, and any one of the myriad of games we had managed to smuggle into the car: Monopoly, Yum, Rumoli, Hi-Q, checkers, chess, not to mention the numerous decks of cards. When cabin fever loomed, Dad would suggest a trip out to the "main drag." Mom was content to go off on her own, browsing around the gift shops. Dad would wander around, most often finding someone with whom to strike up a conversation. Barry and I would happily be left to our own devices in the pinball arcade, tempted to spend more of our allowance than was wise, leaving less for other day trips to nearby Southampton, Port Elgin, Tobermory, or Owen Sound.

Yet the leisure of those two weeks could sometimes elude Mom. If she did not retreat to bed, she would lie for hours behind cotton-balled eyes on the beach. I used to think she just liked to sun herself, and the moist pieces of cotton simply prevented her eyelids from burning. I now wonder how often it was much more than that: a way to mask the depression as it crept up on her. Although Mom cannot swim, when smooth waters permitted, she was known to wade out beyond the third sandbar where she'd float and float until a passing boat unfurled a rolling wave. In retrospect, her aimless passage of time upon the waters of Lake Huron may well have constituted an attempt to escape into her own little world. Sadly, neither the relaxation of being there, nor the boat rides that she so loved were tonic enough to alleviate the rapidly rising doldrums. Over the years, her profound sadness is repeatedly captured through the lens of Dad's camera. Looking back on photos now, it is obvious she was not well. Yet still she struggled, forcing herself through the pain. The tidal wave of depression was simply too powerful for her to rise above.

[AUGUST, LATE 1960s] *Bingo Night at the Sauble Beach Pavilion. Straining my ears to catch the caller's next number under the "b." Above the shuffling of the white ping-pong balls, hearing instead words that alarm me. Mom is quietly confiding in Mary Strathmore, a friend from a nearby cottage, that if it weren't for us kids, Dad would have left years ago. My head spins like those tiny caged balls . . .*

As the dragonfly symphony drifted in through the pavilion windows, barely audible above the din of carefree cottagers, the frail security of my childhood innocence was in part stripped away that warm summer evening. I was embarrassed and ashamed that our family troubles had been exposed. Granted, Mrs. Strathmore knew that something was not quite right with Mom, because there were the brilliant summer days when she would stay in bed, unable to join in with the things our two families did together. But to hear those words come out of Mom's mouth was devastating. I was also racked with guilt. First, for hearing something to which I probably shouldn't have been privy; secondly, because it registered in me that Dad was sacrificing himself for us.

My young mind interpreted those words to mean all the arguing between he and Mom was our fault. If he left, there would be no more fighting. But he stayed because of Barry and me. It was our fault he was unhappy. As much as I hated the arguing between my parents, there had always been the security of Dad's presence. Though Mom's being there was never guaranteed for more than a few months at a time before she'd have to be hospitalized again, day after day, Dad was there. And until that bingo-hall bombshell was dropped in my lap, I had never thought of him going anywhere. What if he did leave one day? Would that be our fault too? What would happen to Mom? To us kids? Amidst periodic cries of "bingo" throughout the hall, I made up my mind to be the very best daughter I could. I'd take care of Barry, look after Mom and do more things around the house to help Dad out, so he wouldn't want to leave. After all, I couldn't think of anybody who had only one parent.

In a way, I had already assumed a caregiving role of sorts, as living with a depressed parent predisposes children to take on added responsibility, or even become parents prematurely within their own family structure. Unfortunately, it was a role for which I was ill-prepared. Under the guise of being a "good little girl," waves of loneliness and fear thrashed within me, drowning the carefree pleasures of childhood.

[AUGUST 1994] Excitement oozes in the voice of our 7-year-old neighbour Louise, as she shares plans for her forthcoming week at summer day camp. It is refreshing to hear such pure anticipation in her voice; I catch myself wondering if I was ever that happy. My memory is jaded with the reels of sadness. While talking to Louise later in the week, I sense that her balloon has deflated. For some undisclosed reason, camp was not all she had dreamed it would be. My heart goes out to her, as I relate to this heavier emotion more readily.

As for my own day camp odyssey, I recall the pit in my stomach every morning as Dad prepared Barry and me to go over to the makeshift campground at Chedoke Hospital. Even years later as my running route took me past the deserted camp, my stomach twinged as I recalled the dread that would set in the night before. How I hated to wave goodbye to Dad in the mornings after we stepped out of the car. Barry and I were usually among the first campers there, so that Dad could get to work on time. I remember that we were attending camp not only because our close friends Elaine and Brian were going, but because Mom was not well and we needed somewhere to go for those two weeks. All the kids except me seemed to be having a good time. I felt alone and out of place, too shy to make friends with the others; even Barry seemed to be fitting in better than I. The experience was made worse because two of the counsellors were also our babysitters: they knew more intimate details of our family problems than I cared to imagine.

The days dragged on; 5:00 p.m. could not come soon enough. What if Dad never came back to get us? That cloud of uncertainty followed me from the craft classes, to the swimming lessons, to the end of the day sing-alongs. It danced overhead, mocking my role as the older sister entrusted with the care of my younger brother. While on the one hand, day camp took us away from our bedridden mother, and the need to play in hushed tones around the house, it was, on the other hand, as if being away from home projected me into a world that reinforced my insecurity and place in the world; something just never felt right about spending nine hours a day engaged in complicated Popsicle-stick crafts and songs I had no voice to sing: Who would be there to watch over Mom?

In 1978, Dad decided we'd try something different for our annual summer vacation. After weeks of meticulous planning through CAA, Dad drove us down into the eastern United States, through New York, West Virginia, Tennessee, New Hampshire, and Pennsylvania. Having never been anywhere besides the Lake Huron environs, Barry and I were eager to explore this new territory. Dad had carefully planned the itinerary: Whiteface Mountain, Lake Placid, Ausable Chasm, Hershey Chocolate Factory, Amish Country, Corning Glass

Company, even winery tours he thought Mom would enjoy. Yet despite the breathtaking beauty of the Adirondack Mountains and rolling patchwork countryside, Mom slipped deeper and deeper into a depression throughout the course of the trip. Much as she tried to satisfy Dad's efforts and her kids' hopes for a fun time, it was fruitless. It was all she could do to get herself from the motel room to the car before we headed off to the next state. The years of defeated summer holidays had taken their toll. Dad swore we would never take another family trip again. I should have known it would be but a matter of time before he cracked, but at 16, I was too preoccupied with my own hairline fractures beneath the surface to notice ...

Thirteen: Road to self-destruction

Supertramp's "Hide in your Shell" throbs through my body and fills my mind as quickly as the vodka and orange juice. Gradually, the parameters of the room lose shape, faces of friends contort, and dizziness washes over. Oblivious to the voices around me, I make my way out of the house, down the street, around the corner, and into Calhoun Park, where I slump into the cool grass, beneath the stares of the stars, succumbing to the comfort of nothingness . . .

THE LONG-TERM effect of a parent's depression manifests itself in many, often hidden, ways. I will never forget the August afternoon in 1994, when, in a rare emotional reference to the past, Dad emphatically stated, "You two coped better than most kids — always did as you were told." I was taken aback, for I have never conceived of myself as coping well during Mom's down times. On the surface, it may have appeared as if we were, but that was situational coping: doing chores around the house, not misbehaving or asking for things. We may have even coped beyond our years, as roles and responsibilities shifted in response to the needs of the family. From an early age, instinct dictated the need to be a caretaker of sorts not only for my brother, but also for my parents. Mom needed to be cared for like a child because she was sick. Dad needed constant monitoring of his perpetually volatile temper.

[OCTOBER 17, 1978 — JOURNAL ENTRY] *Dad is in a real shitty mood, and Mom's been crying. I was trying to help her figure out how to use the new washing machine before Dad came down, but I'm not sure how it's supposed to work. She's sad just thinking that she bought it with some of the money from Grandma Bonner's estate. Dad comes down and starts arguing with Mom about how to use it — he has no patience whatsoever. I sort of talked back to him ... I don't know why he always gets so temperamental. "Everybody's on my back," he yelled. "Maybe I'll just pack up my bags and get the hell out!" He always says that though. One of these days I'm gonna let right into him and then we'll both be sorry. I hope Mom doesn't get another one of her spells again because of this ...*

Up until my mid-teens, I endeavoured to handle Mom's cycles of depression in ways I can now see were constructive: by creating an almost shrine-like atmosphere of comfort and security in my bedroom. Surrounded by books, portable record player, and an assortment of collectibles, I tried to block out whatever was happening beyond my door. I always wished I could do something to make Mom better and my parents stop arguing. Failing that, by about the age of 10 or 12, I adopted my Grandma Bonner's yen for rearranging my bedroom furniture, discovering that doing so at least gave me a sense of control over my own space. Once, when Mom was sick and Dad was at work, I boldly went out to buy wallpaper and a carpet for my bedroom with money I'd saved from two part-time jobs I held after school. Despite thinking I could be in trouble for doing so, I was driven by a defiant voice that assured me I deserved it, spending as much time in my bedroom as I did. Altering my physical space was a way to cocoon me from the rest of my family. Channelling energy into physical acts helped redirect thoughts and keep my own simmering issues on the back burner. Whenever the contents neared boiling, I'd tighten the lid to smother whatever threatened to surface within, escaping reality and gradually isolating myself from those closest to me. How much pressure could have been relieved by engaging in the present-day version of a support group for teens troubled by mentally ill parents! Had that been the case, I might have had the courage to contact Kate, the girl I'd known from public school, whose father also suffered from clinical depression. Instead, I only wrote in my journal when Mom told me the awful news about a man I had never met, and whose daughter I only slightly knew.

[DECEMBER 5, 1978 — JOURNAL ENTRY] *Kate's dad is dead. Poor man committed suicide today — gassed himself to death in his garage. Mom used to work with him at the Hydro years ago. She said that he was so quiet and nice, but always seemed troubled. My heart goes out to Kate so much because God knows how many times the thoughts about Mom doing the same thing have gone through my head. When she's down, I always think and shudder about that. God bless Kate and her family. I sympathize with them so much . . .*

At the time of her father's death, Kate and I were attending different high schools. I didn't have the courage to contact her, though it would not have been difficult to look her up. After all, what would I have said? When we crossed paths again two years later in Grade 13, I wanted to reach out somehow, to acknowledge her pain. Periodically, in the cafeteria or in the hallway, I would catch myself watching her, wondering what life for her was like now. How did she concentrate on school? How was she able to cope without her father? All of my questions and thoughts went unanswered. I felt terribly guilty. After all, my Mom was still alive.

Alive or dead — there were times when I didn't know which was better. It was for that reason that my Dad's armchair theory on coping he presented that August day in 1994 resonated emptiness within me: how distant he was from his own flesh and blood. There is indeed a marked evolution from the lost carefreeness of childhood to the increasingly reckless teenage and adult years. Though it was never drawn to our family's attention, my brother and I were almost certainly depressed children. Typically, childhood depression is characterized by those who are shy, withdrawn, experience changes in sleep and appetite, and harbour feelings of worthlessness or guilt about parents' arguing and illness, sometimes to the point of wanting to run away or kill themselves. Such children are also vulnerable to substance abuse as a way of coping with the emotional inner turmoil, and all the signs and symptoms point to Barry and me being typical of such troubled teens.

During the tenth grade, in 1978, as the revolving door of Mom's depression kept whirling us around, another door opened, seducing me along the road to self-destruction. The door was passed through innocently enough, with the inevitable teenage forays into the world of underage drinking and secretive smoking — cigarettes and other-wise. But it was a door through which I would not go gently, or be able to close. From the age of 16, few were the safe-haven detours I allowed myself, preferring the long and winding road to self-abuse, as weekend staples of alcohol, cigarettes, marijuana and "soft drugs" took over my life. For reasons unclear at that time, I embraced mood-altering substances with a passion that surpassed the others in my group of friends. Changing my bedroom furniture around no longer did the trick.

There was neither a badge of honour nor sympathy awarded for waking with my first bona fide hangover, confined to bed with an ice pack, claiming I had fallen on the ice getting out of a friend's car. Coming home drunk more times than I can recall, Barry sneaking into my room to clean up after me. My head hanging over the side of the bed, making a valiant effort to aim for the white enamel pan with the red trim he had thoughtfully come running upstairs with. Heaving with a violence, I promised some faceless god I'd never do it again. The room reeked of a ghastly combination of alcohol and cigarettes, creating a nauseating centrifugal force inside my head. Vaguely aware of Barry urging me to put one of my feet on the floor to ground me, while he kept the radio on low for me through the night. How many times we hurried to each other's bedside sensing the call of duty in the wee hours of the morning after umpteen drinking binges. We were partners in crime, as our parents surely lay knowingly across the hall.

Somehow, my escapades of the night before were seldom brought into serious question by either one of my parents. Even when I came in noticeably drunk, having first passed out in Calhoun Park after leaving a party and then being delivered home by friends, Dad said nothing. Whether he just did not have the energy, because there were more important things to worry about with Mom being sick, he simply came in my room, sat on the edge of my bed and hugged me. From that point on, years of contrived stories and white lies permitted me to explore the many avenues of substance use and abuse without significant parental challenge. In a strange twist of psychology that I could never figure out, Dad began chiding me, even around friends, in an oddly jesting manner, for drinking and being drunk — even when I wasn't. Consciously or unconsciously, I learned to take advantage of Mom's sickness, and took for granted her easy-going nature when she was well. But for every time I thought I was getting away with it, I was fooling nobody more than myself.

Early on in the tenth grade, I had developed a rapport with Mrs. Michaels, an English teacher whose class I was in for two consecutive years. Perhaps in my own mind, I conceived our relationship to extend beyond the confines of grammar rules and Shakespearean sonnets. Her casual and easy-going nature was conducive to considerably relaxed teacher–student dynamics. My circle of friends played up to her fondness for joking with me and teasing about my predisposition to blushing. As I became more withdrawn at home, distressed by Mom's frequent depressions and angered by Dad's constant arguing with her, my spirits were always lifted by the daily bantering with Mrs. Michaels. She was radiant. She was life. She was everything in contrast to home, where it was gloomy and lifeless. Day after day, this woman was there, showing an interest in me in a way that no adult ever had. How I wished she could whisk me away in the little olive green Ford Mustang she drove daily to school. Yet as our conversing took on an even more amiable tone, the more I struggled to subdue a rising confusion within me. By the fall of 1978, the daughter my Dad believed had always coped well was doing anything but, as a sampling of journal entries and acting-out behaviour over a particularly anxious six-month period will attest.

[SEPTEMBER 17, 1978 — JOURNAL ENTRY] *Dull day today. Exactly how I feel. Pouring rain. I'm getting these awful pains in my stomach, even if I'm just sitting. I think it's being eaten away . . .*

[OCTOBER 3, 1978 — JOURNAL ENTRY] *Fuck day. Fuck everyone. Dad, Barry, even poor Mom and my friends are getting on my nerves. At lunch, I thought I was going to explode, I felt so out of place. Just wanted to go home, flop on the bed and turn the stereo up full blast . . .*

Through Grade 11, my reputation as an "alky" and a "stoner" spread beyond my circle of friends as drinking episodes escalated from passing out at weekend parties to occasional classroom drunkenness.

[OCTOBER 27, 1978] *Pre-meditated lunch hour drinking alone . . . up at my third-floor locker, pouring the beer that I'd pilfered from the fridge that morning into a Coke can, not caring that Mrs. Michaels is in the classroom behind me. She comes out and asks what I'm doing. I look suspicious, she says. Nothing, I mumble, averting my eyes, a strange mix of relief and anxiety that she has seen me. She doesn't pursue it but watches me with a quizzical half smile as I squirm past her and down the stairs. Through the crowded cafeteria, not stopping to speak with my friends who call out to me. I wave absently over at their table and keep going out the back door. Across the parking lot, and along the path beyond the track. Suddenly stooping down to oblige an obsessive compulsion to pick up pieces of broken glass. Putting them in my pocket. Voices faintly behind me. Jenny and Danielle, I recognize as they come closer. Alarmed at what they see. Blood on my hands. I don't feel a thing — and don't know why I am doing it. Late for biology class. Stumbling in with glassy eyes and a dopey expression. People stare and giggle. Time to work on the cats. Normally repulsed, I boldly pick up the dead, skinned animal with my bare hands, unfazed by the feel of its cold, clammy flesh and the burning stench of formaldehyde . . .*

While classmates and acquaintances thought my behaviour was funny and pretty cool, my closest friends, including the loyal partners in crime, Peigi and Wendy, couldn't understand why I was drinking to excess and making such scenes — both in and out of school. I could offer no reasonable explanation. Nor could I be bothered to find one.

[NOVEMBER 26, 1978 — JOURNAL ENTRY] *Feel pretty shitty. Don't know why. Just don't feel like talking to anybody. Just want to stay in my room and veg out. Dad, Mom, and Barry are all pissed off at me. They say I'm acting snotty lately. Probably true but lately I don't really care. Get grouchy even when they ask me a question. Glad to get out of the house . . .*

[DECEMBER 9, 1978 — JOURNAL ENTRY] *Something going on inside me and I'm not hungry hardly. I love it because I'm not eating that much but it feels weird. Really bad pains again in the middle of my stomach . . .*

With Christmas approaching, my gloom and general irritability was at least understandable; our family has always dreaded holiday season, because more often than not, Mom faded out of the picture at some point — if she was ever in it to begin with.

[DECEMBER 22, 1978 — JOURNAL ENTRY] *I'm feeling pretty depressed. Maybe because I've got this awful feeling Mom is slipping again. Every night I pray she won't. It's just murder around here whenever she gets one of her spells. I'm really worried. If she does, I'm at the point where I'm sick and tired of it happening at least once every year. I mean, I can't understand why it has to be our family. Jesus, I hope I'm wrong . . .*

93

Though I seldom sensed incorrectly, that year, I was premature in my prediction.

[DECEMBER 25, 1978 — JOURNAL ENTRY] *Excellent day. My best Christmas present was that Mom isn't sick. I couldn't ask for anything better, believe me! Must have only been one of her bilious headaches that was making her seem down. So thankful Mom is okay. Waiting for right chance to tell her about my best "present"...*

Though 1978 ended on a positive note, any resolutions about cleaning up my own act in the new year were quickly dashed.

[JANUARY 9, 1979 — JOURNAL ENTRY] *Depressed when I got up, so had vodka and orange juice before I left for school. Felt better when I got there. Came home and felt depressed again. Mom is really slipping this time I think. Get out. Walk over to San Pharmacy to pick up pills for her.*

[JANUARY 10, 1979 — JOURNAL ENTRY] *Super tired all the time. Can hardly stay awake in my classes. Susan thinks I'm being rude! Think I'll try the Coke and aspirins before I go to school today. Supposed to give you a high. Something's gotta work...*

With the second semester of Grade 11 fast approaching, my ever-changing moods and mind-altering drinking were consistently interfering with school.

[JANUARY 17, 1979 — JOURNAL ENTRY] *I think I am setting a record for lates and absences. Feel so lazy. Head throbbing from all this mess in my mind. Don't know how Mom can cope with having a headache every day, which she says she does. Then again, have to give her credit for being alive most of the time ...*

[JANUARY 21, 1979 — JOURNAL ENTRY] *Drank my beer way too fast last night and thought I was going to have to bring it up for sure. After I drank it, I just lay there in the dark with the radio on low. Wish I didn't have to go to school tomorrow . . . or do anything for that matter . . .*

My grades slipped, particularly in English, when I ended up with Mrs. Michaels as my teacher again in the eleventh grade. Having been an "A" student of hers the previous year, my slump to the mid "Cs" only validated there was more to the mark than met the eye. I remained distracted and withdrawn, unable to participate in class for fear of bringing attention to myself, convinced my turmoil was transparent.

Though I harboured a desire to speak with Mrs. Michaels more candidly than any other teacher, or even my closest friends, about what was going on inside of me, I became increasingly nervous and tongue-tied, heart beating in time to the sweat forming beneath my clothes. I was emotionally vulnerable, and absorbed every nuance of our daily conversations. When she innocently made a ribbing comment about my weight, I was devastated. As a broad-shouldered, well-endowed teenager, I was extremely self-conscious about my body at the best of times. Although I carried fewer than 120 pounds on my five-foot-two frame, I began exercising in my bedroom and jogging enough circles around the park to wipe out any calories I'd needlessly consumed during the day. My weight proceeded to plummet until the indicator on the scales hovered just over the 100-pound mark. When I still complained of being fat, my friends Sharon and Elaine both decided I was anorexic and gave me one of the first articles to appear on the topic in magazines like *Miss Chatelaine* and *Seventeen*. Contrary to their fears, I was relieved to be reassured of my relative slightness, and made a mental note to remember that people would notice if I started to "blimp-up" again. While I had neither control over my uncomfortable thoughts and feelings, nor over the miserable situation at home, at least I could exercise control over my weight. For that I was relieved.

On another occasion, Mrs. Michaels confronted me, with the usual twinkle in her eyes, about being "different" from my other friends. The innuendo was overpowering. I was all the more paranoid because in one of my classes, we were discussing Oedipus and Electra, and the Freudian complexities of father-daughter-mother relationships. I was secretly hoping there was nothing in my subconscious I was sublimating: it was all too weird for me. But I could not help but wonder if my anxiety around Mrs. Michaels was somehow related to Mom being sick. Was I attracted to her for what was lacking in my relationship with my Mom? Was it that she represented a reliable motherly figure for me? Was I betraying the woman who gave birth to me by being so attached to another? Or was Mrs. Michaels appealing to something deeper and more conflicted inside of me?

I was confused, ashamed, guilt-ridden, and afraid. The thoughts in my head were explosive; I wanted to crawl into a bomb-shelter and die. It was quicker to drink instead. Drinking blocked things out by drowning feelings that were swimming forcefully to the surface. I began drinking before and during school, often going out of my way to do so, particularly when I knew there was a risk of Mrs. Michaels catching me.

[FEBRUARY 2, 1979] *Down into fruit cellar while Dad is taking his 6:45 a.m. shower. Pouring Beefeater gin into the thermos, adding Canada Dry tonic until it is full. Careful to top up the perpetually marked gin bottle with water. Lunchtime swigging of my private stock in the girls' washroom. Out for a walk then into English class. Head too heavy to hold up. Din of friends whispering around me, trying to wake me up before Mrs. Michaels notices. But she never seems to miss a single move of mine. She's standing over me. I cannot rise to the occasion of meeting her eyes. After class, she holds me back. She looks deep into my eyes that cannot stay focused on her. No explanation I can offer though I am screaming inside. She leads me by the arm down to the office. "Oh God no. Please don't," I plead. Didn't expect her to do this. Class change-over. People watching, as I attempt to wiggle away from her grasp. Spot Jenny by her locker. Call out for her to help me. She's crying, "What are you doing, Nancy?" Into the office. Mrs. Michaels' voice from somewhere, then she's gone, leaving me alone with the formidable Miss Chattell, the vice-principal. Surprisingly calm while she questions me about what happened. She wants to call my Mom. Go ahead, I think, she won't answer the phone anyway. When Miss Chattell finally hangs up after what seems an eternity, I mumble that I'm just tired because I've lost weight and haven't been sleeping properly. The Oscar is mine. She grants me permission to go home. Mom is up getting a cracker. When she sees me she cries. Thinks something is wrong with me. Worried I'm getting too skinny. Never dawns on her I'm drunk.*

At home, Dad, Mom, and Barry were all noticing my increasing list-lessness, remarking that I didn't seem to care about things anymore. Their comments only pushed me further away, for I hated my life and myself.

Reading back over the journals I began keeping in high school has been a disquieting journey. It has also shed light on the patterns that emerged and solidified as I internalized emotions and sought to escape Mom's recurring depression, my parents' incessant fighting, and my own burgeoning inner conflict that dared not speak its name — for to do so in the 1970s would have been to commit virtual social suicide.

   Though I managed to leave Sir Allan MacNab High School in June 1980 with a diploma in hand, I never left behind the most com-pelling forces of destruction, nor the feelings for the woman who triggered them.

Fourteen: Ten-cent solution

[AUGUST 1980] *Sneaking out on to the 14th floor balcony of the hotel. Daring to smoke the first of the Marlboro cigarettes I'd managed to purchase from the machine in the lobby. Inhaling both the salty breeze off the Pacific Ocean below me and the bittersweet nicotine, my head spins ...*

IN THE SUMMER after my high school graduation, Mom and I took a trip to Hawaii: the destination of her dreams. Over the years, I'd always felt sorry for Mom, because so many people she knew went on holidays to Florida or Jamaica. Dad hated flying, so he didn't care if Mom went with me. We used some of the money left to her when Grandma Bonner passed away two years prior. Mom was really looking forward to it, and we were set to have the time of our lives.

We stayed at the opulent (to us) Miramar Hotel, next to the International Market Place, where we would wander for breakfasts of succulent pineapple, melon and other tropical delicacies. Later in the day, between Mai-Tais and Chi-Chis by the pool or down at the beach, we made our way through the streets of Waikiki and around the island of Oahu. Looking back at the photos taken with my trusty Kodak Instamatic camera, I am jarred by the sick look in Mom's eyes in most of them. I now appreciate how desperately she was forcing herself to make the most of that long-awaited journey into paradise. Some days, Mom would sleep in a little longer than usual. It was then I would make my bold move out to the balcony for the guilt-ridden smoke.

Guilty on two counts: for smoking behind Mom's back, and for taking advantage of the extra time she was staying in bed. My gut told me something was wrong, but I discarded worry in favour of that private indulgence.

My indiscretions took me beyond the balcony to the seedy side streets of Waikiki. Early on in the trip, I was naively charmed by the flashy smile and beach-bum good looks of a fellow on the hotel staff. With Mom seemingly content to watch TV for the evening, I joined him and his friends for a party on the town. Before night fell, the drugs came out. I popped the little blue pill they offered and washed it down with a Budweiser, as the locals were not Chi-Chi drinkers. Then the greenest pot ("Maui-Wowee" they told me) I'd ever seen took me higher and higher. I became incredibly stoned and paranoia engulfed me. We ended up at a restaurant, where I became increasingly convinced they were concocting an elaborate scheme to leave me with the bill or plotting to have me smuggle dope back to Canada. Without warning, I fled the restaurant, flagged a cab, and somehow made it safely back to the hotel, where Mom slept unknowingly. If anything had happened to me, I can't imagine how Mom would have coped. She depended on me entirely during that trip. By throwing caution to the wind and flirting with fate, I had put my life in jeopardy and abdicated my responsibility as daughter-cum-caretaker.

The taste of the Hawaiian tropics lingered two weeks later when I entered Southmount Secondary, one of only two public schools in Hamilton where Grade 13 was offered at that time. I was in my glory, as weekend parties were frequent and fostered a freedom to increase alcohol use while fearlessly expanding my repertoire of recreational drugs to include hashish and amphetamines. I also acquired a party buddy and confidante by the name of Leanne, who would prove to be a loyal friend through many dispirited phases to follow. All the while I was increasingly tuned out to the stress at home. Whereas my foray into substance use and abuse remained a silent and uncontested struggle, Dad's more overt, direct response to his own issues was an explosive nightmare for me.

[SPRING 1981] *Dad drives me down the Hamilton mountain to my Red Cross Lifesaving class, via the route commonly known as the Jolley Cut Access. All of a sudden, he bursts out that he wishes he could just drive off the edge. I stiffen; the blood drains downward. We hadn't yet covered this in the weekly Red Cross class. But surely I am dreaming. With only a few minutes until we reach our destination, I manage to ask what he means by that, terrified of his response. It then comes pouring out, how fed up he is with life: "I just can't do it anymore." As if reading my mind, he added that he probably wouldn't do anything because of "you kids." I climb out of the car in a daze. It flashes through my mind that I may never see him again. . .*

Ever since the "bingo hall bombshell" in the late 1960s, Barry and I were often reminded of Dad's enormous sense of responsibility to stay with the family for our sake. In that split second as he drove me down the mountain, it became horribly clear that in honouring this commitment, he had been pushed to the brink. After so many years of being on the alert for Mom taking some desperate action, my suicide watch was instantly forced to expand. How could I not have known Dad was that despondent? The fear my Dad would commit the ultimate act was intensified by the thought that he might attempt to put the whole family out of our misery. God knows he had every reason. Since the time I was born, he had sacrificed himself for the sake of his family. Whatever did he get in return? He had not asked for a depressive wife anymore than he'd planned on a son who fled Hamilton at the age of 17 or a withdrawn daughter like me. That night in the car convinced me he too could be pushed over the edge as easily as Mom. Both my parents had to be protected from the core of their daughter at all cost. And it would be a high price to pay — for all of us . . .

Despite the toll of excessive substance abuse on my high school study habits, my grades were deemed worthy of acceptance to McMaster, my hometown university. In September 1981, on the threshold of post-secondary academia, I readied myself for a reprieve from the destructive tendencies within. In hindsight, the campus, nestled in the west-end of the city, offered a security and a certain anonymity that appealed to my need to escape, and the library once again became my second home. University was also a place where I began uncovering the bohemian spirit that longed to break free. But I was still caught in an insidious web of striving to be the dutiful daughter, as the delicate life threads around Mom's neck became increasingly taut; a slip-noose attached to a rusted anchor.

[APRIL 1982 — JOURNAL ENTRY] *Mom and Dad's Caribbean cruise. Dad had one hell of a time and Mom — well, next to Hawaii it's something she's always dreamed of. But she has been in bed for the 14 days they've been home. Shit damn! Mom's Aunt Annie died last week and Mom didn't even flinch. It's a mean episode this time. She's lost 12 pounds in two weeks and collapsed three times in three days. Was almost overdosing on pills. She relies so much on those goddamned shock treatments — can she really not help herself? Who knows? Dr. Simpson threatens not to administer any more treatments after this set is over. "She's got to help herself!" he ruthlessly admonishes us in the same slap-in-the-face manner he's been brandishing toward Mom for years. Want to run for my own sanity, but know that won't solve anything. Now trying to write first-year exams. I was a nervous wreck for sociology final. I'd only studied five hours and cried almost all day. Leanne has been a real true-blue friend. Always there when I need to talk or just get out. Such a vicious circle. Will it ever end?*

What I really wondered was, who would reach the end first?

[MARCH 1982 — JOURNAL ENTRY] *Oh dear God. Johnnie Hayworth is dead. Suicide at age 15. Why such a guy? Beautiful smile, wavy brown hair, a quiet, friendly boy. Shattered everybody, even people like me who had only met him a few times through Leanne. I cried when she told me. What a damn shame. What does it feel like when it gets that bad?*

[JUNE 22, 1982 — JOURNAL ENTRY] *Well, I almost did it. Almost sent myself over the brink. Have been abusing myself to no end, physically, mentally and emotionally. It's like I'm two different people. Working over 50 hours a week between Jean Junction clothing store and Jackson Square movie theatre since writing last exam in April. Hardly sleeping, going out drinking, losing weight, smoking (both) and just going wild with diet pills and bennies to get me through history night class. Waking Monday with panicky feeling I didn't want to go to work. Invaded with paranoia that people know about me. Need to get my head settled. All I need is some time. For all this family has been through, I'm damn lucky this never happened to me before. I've been stronger I guess, what with Mom's depressions and all, never really thinking about my own self as much. Now I know I cannot handle it anymore . . .*

[JUNE 24, 1982 — JOURNAL ENTRY] *Still don't know which fucking end is up. What am I putting myself through? I can hardly even speak. Feel as if I'm looking at myself from a distance. Am I hitting rock bottom or what? Haven't even been calling friends back when they call. Can't even finish dialling the numbers. Leanne is the first person I've spoken to in a week; just hearing her voice made me cry. What a friend — even two minutes on the phone elicits a laugh. Wish I could just be taken away to some desert island. Just for a while until I get my head clear. Feel terrible for what this is doing to my family. They don't know what kind of mood to expect from me next. Especially hard on Mom, but can't seem to help it. Time and again, I think of poor Johnnie. What does it feel like to put a bullet through your own head?*

Fifteen: Notes from the edge

[SEPTEMBER 22, 1982] *Mom has fallen. She is so weak from ingesting next to nothing for days on end. She has lost nearly 20 pounds in less than a month. She has even stopped taking her pills. I hear the thud on the floor above me, and race up the stairs, heart pounding in my mouth. She is in a crumpled heap in the hallway just outside the bathroom. I'm terrified. Her scaly skin and dry, foul mouth betray the level of dehydration she has reached. Her body tissues are wasting away, releasing toxic substances into the bloodstream. Her mind is a cloud of dust ...*

By September 1982, Mom's remissions were getting shorter. From once, maybe twice a year, it had been barely three months since her last bout of depression. This time, not even the most recent series of shock treatments were kicking in: she'd already had 19. Was she immune? Or was there nothing left to burn? Having reached the fork in the road, she was careening toward that point of no return ...

After somehow getting Mom back into bed that first day of fall 1982, I called Dad at work to explain what had happened and asked him what I should do. He had reached the end of his tether. He told me to do whatever I wanted, because nothing he said or did made any difference. I could only hang up and sob, agonizing over my duty as a daughter. I didn't even know who else to call, because Mom was in a "limbo" period. That very morning she had been told by our family doctor's secretary that Dr. MacIntosh was not available. She would have to wait for the on-call physician, Dr. Orville Traymore, to get back to her. Hours later, she was still waiting.

To further aggravate things, her psychiatrist, Dr. Simpson, had recently all but washed his hands of her. When I spoke to him earlier in the day, explaining how desperately worried I was about my Mom, he coldly stated that "if she doesn't want to go to the hospital, then tell her to get up out of bed." Period. A heartless ultimatum for a profoundly ill woman. Over the years this was the same man who had become almost a god-like figure to Mom, wielding his "power" to authorize the shock treatments he dealt out like candy. With the cord now severed, Mom understandably felt no one cared. It was, in fact, as if nobody did. She repeatedly uttered things like she wished she would "just pass on." On that bleak September day, I wondered if she somehow wouldn't be better off.

Ashamed of that thought, I broke all the rules and called Dr. MacIntosh at home. By the time Dr. Traymore called, I feared it would be too late. I desperately tried to impress upon Dr. MacIntosh the urgency of the situation. Surely he would understand. In the 20 years since he had helped my mother give birth to me, I had certainly never been so vocal about anything. Mom was deteriorating and I was alarmed by the intensity of her nothing-left-to-live-for state of mind. I pleaded with him to do something. His words, as I wrote them down that day, are no less appalling now as they were then.

"She has you all on a string. She knows this is a way to get your Dad mad. She knows it will make you feel guilty, sorry for her; she is pulling at your sympathy." He asks me whether Mom falls when she is alone, suggesting that it's nothing but an attention-seeker when she does it otherwise. The only thing he can do is hospitalize her for physical reasons such as dehydration, because he has no authority in the mental health area. *"She's got to help herself,"* he says flatly — as callously as one who tosses a deflated life preserver to a drowning woman. *"I'll tell you right out,"* he continues, *"that yes, one day she will probably self-destruct. She's not a strong person. I've seen it happen so many times, and people ask 'why didn't you do something?' It's a dead-end."*

Over the years, the major stumbling block in securing assistance for Mom, particularly when she reached such dire depths, was that a course of action was highly subjective. Difficult as it was to know how to handle and support Mom during those episodes, unless she was deemed to be in imminent danger to herself or others, we were given the emotional run-around by doctors who claimed their hands were tied by the Mental Health Act of the time. I hate to think what would have happened if Dr. MacIntosh had not finally relented and come to the house later that afternoon. Standing in the shadows of the bathroom, I numbly listened to their conversation.

Dr. MacIntosh is badgering Mom into a corner. Her deep, defensive tone of response is one I've never heard. He is quizzing her about her interests; telling her maybe she should go back to work because she wasn't like this when she had a job. Mom emphatically says that she was, even when she worked briefly as a volunteer for the Lung Association. He then assails her with guilt. He suggests that being sick is a way to get back at my Dad, but by doing so she is hurting Barry and me even more. "I've never seen or heard your little girl so upset," he goads her. She cries, and in a weak and withered voice, she tries to explain that she has a constant headache, except when she is in bed. "It's because of the arguing," she weeps. Dr. MacIntosh then infers that if Dad is the cause, then Mom should leave him. She hollowly replies that she has nowhere to go, to which he responds "then get him out." I am shocked by the way he is rubbing salt in the wound of my parents' already fragile relationship. He is manipulating her, toying with her emotions.

Dr. MacIntosh's constant barrage finally forces Mom to get up to eat and drink something, the threat of hospitalization hanging over her head. She calls to me. She tells me she doesn't want to go back into the hospital again. She has had enough. She is crying like a poor soul because she can't open the frozen orange juice can. Her trembling and weakened hands fall to her sides in despair. Sobbing, she suddenly says she wants to go and look around the stores. After her first meal in weeks, half a cup of Old South orange juice, a quarter cup of Special K cereal, and a shot-glass portion of milk, Dr. MacIntosh encourages her to take a bath. Mom says she will after she lies down.

He presses on: "Why don't you stay up and do the dishes or something to make yourself feel worthwhile?" I cringe at his dispassionate tone. Mom has no answer other than she will lie down first. I want to shake her, yell at her, comfort her. She is yawning, even though she has been in bed for three weeks. Literally. Dr. MacIntosh cannot believe it when I say that she does not eat with us, nor does she come out to watch TV. I realize with a sinking feeling that he has absolutely no concept of what Mom is experiencing, or what we endure as a family, even though he has been her doctor since before I was born.

When Dad finally arrived home from work, the drama intensified. Dr. MacIntosh escalated the tension by telling him that Mom just couldn't cope with his bark anymore; she was fed up. "She's got something against you, Henry," Dr. MacIntosh is needling.

"Why the hell do I bother doing things around here then?" Dad shouts. My heart throbs in my mouth. "Might as well put a bullet through her head," he yells in a tone that chills me to the bone.

Dad's vicious words, laced with homicidal venom, sliced the stale air and hung like a premature skeleton in our midst ...

wherein lies the answer

the true meaning of helplessness
watching someone you love die
no words have meaning
no gestures have strength
you silently watch her slip
into that deep, dark, empty space
and faith in tomorrow
becomes a vain prayer for no more
will this be the end
you dare to wonder
is this what her life
was meant to become
is this the fate
for which she was destined
or is it only the beginning
of her new life beyond
one which shall know
neither sorrow, nor angst
nor the weight of depression
nor the horror of the shock
only the sky, ever blue to be touched . . .

Part II: Starting from scratch

Sixteen: Now or never

[OCTOBER 9, 1982 — JOURNAL ENTRY] *At this point in my life, I realize that I am not a very happy person. I mean, what exactly do I have going for me? Mom is in the psychiatric ward of St. Joseph's; Dad is on my case about trivial things; I'm incredibly far behind in school; my personal feelings are severely disoriented. Keep thinking about Mom and how this home life is going to continue. It is a vicious circle. What does the future hold for poor Mom? Dear God, please help these new doctors find some answer. It rips me apart, no matter how much I want to run. I'm torn in between. What if she really can't help herself? Is there ever an end?*

SOMETIME BETWEEN Wednesday, September 22, and Saturday, October 9, 1982, Mom was admitted to Hamilton's St. Joseph's Hospital, under the care of a new psychiatrist. It was the last hope.

St. Joseph's seemed to be an odd choice of institutions for Mom. I think it had something to do with the portraits of nuns that graced the walls and the various religious icons strategically placed throughout the building. Although the psychiatric wing of St. Joe's was not quite as sterile and reeking of despair as the Henderson Hospital, where Mom had been incarcerated numerous times over the years, it was an archaic institution that exuded a chilling oppression. There was also a foreboding apprehension about this hospitalization: it was the end of the line as we knew it.

Through a side entrance and past an inappropriately dismal obstetric ward, I would make my way up the stairs to the second floor, to the unit where all comings and goings were strictly monitored and visitors were required to sign in and out. Privacy was a definite commodity. With the nursing "guard" station positioned right in view of the elevators, staff and whoever else cared to look witnessed any last-minute tears and hugs. Uncomfortable as it was to engage in such public displays of affection, I knew it was important for them to see that this woman was loved. She deserved to be well treated. She was somebody. She was my Mom.

Once in St. Joe's, Mom was under the care of Dr. Morley Reimer. Well respected in the field of psychiatry, he had a very methodical and no-nonsense approach to patient care. The first couple of weeks in St. Joseph's Hospital were hell on Mom. In order to do an accurate assessment of her physical and mental condition, she was subject to a virtual detoxification. For the first time in 20 years, her body was medication free, and she endured a withdrawal state not unlike that of an alcoholic or heroin addict. After Dr. Reimer's initial assessment of Mom, he suspected she would be a good candidate for lithium carbonate, a naturally occurring, simple white powder found in mineral water and rocks, quite similar in substance to table salt.

Discovered in the 19th century, it was not until the late 1940s that lithium was first found to have calming, curative properties useful for the treatment of mania. Gradually, it became recognized for its ability to alter neurotransmitters in a manner similar to the antidepressant, tranquilizer, and electroshock therapies of the 1950s and 1960s. Although lithium carbonate is now heralded as a great equalizer for manic depression (also referred to as bipolar disorder), it is not as widely prescribed for those with unipolar disorders (depression) like Mom. Although lithium regulates mood swings, both manic and depressive states, it is not by the same token a cure. And it is not without potentially dangerous side effects. Despite its basal composition, lithium carbonate is a potent drug that affects the body's plasma. Regular blood tests are necessary to strictly monitor the lithium levels in the body. Unlike antidepressants and tranquilizers, the prescribed dosage of lithium is within a similar range for most people. The lowest dose possible is optimum, as the risk of toxicity and the effect on certain organs is reduced. The more common side effects of lithium pertain to the thyroid (hypothyroidism), the heart (altered EKG patterns), vision (fluid build-up in the eye ducts), neurological disturbances (tremors, gait and speech impairment, altered concentration and energy), and the kidneys. Because lithium is excreted through the kidneys, those tissues are vulnerable to inflammation during the filtration process. If the damage is deemed or projected to be severe, lithium is no longer an option.

Such was the case with my Mom in 1979, when she was first tested for lithium compatibility. At that time, the results indicated there was a 99 percent chance her kidneys would be adversely affected, and she would probably have to be on dialysis for the rest of her life. Faced with the lesser of two evils, the lithium avenue was dismissed by Dr. Simpson. That another psychiatrist was advocating lithium treatment fewer than three years later sure didn't make much sense to us laypeople. Who were we to believe? Had we been previously misled by Dr. Simpson — or worse, were we not getting the full picture now from the "esteemed" Dr. Reimer?

Nevertheless, after several weeks of rigorous testing at St. Joe's, Mom was deemed an ideal candidate for lithium. Whether her body chemistry had altered significantly, or whether more thorough investigation was conducted, we never knew what accounted for such an apparently radical shift in Mom's body composition. Then again, it was commonplace for us to be in the dark about matters concerning Mom's health. About the only thing we did know was that in order to keep recurring depressions at bay, she would have to be on lithium for the rest of her life. In other words, this was it. No more dilly-dallying around with other medications. No more ECT. But with a sinking realization, we knew that if the lithium didn't work, nothing would.

Altogether, Mom spent close to two months in the psychiatric ward of St. Joseph's Hospital that fall of 1982. During that time, visits to her were strained under the weight of whatever veiled optimism we could muster. Mom seemed pleased with Dr. Reimer. Though the light of her life had been rapidly extinguishing, under his care, there was a power surge of hope. Toward the end of her stay, we learned that Mom was responding favourably to the lithium, and would need to be constantly monitored while taking it: in other words, forever, if things went the way Dr. Reimer led her to believe. In conjunction with the lithium, Mom was also to take Parnate, an antidepressant in the MAO inhibitor family, which also required dietary restrictions. The list of foods to curtail, or have only in moderation, was daunting, but she'd have to manage.

Seventeen: Walking wounded

"Days of absence, sad and dreary,
Clothed in sorrow's dark array, —
Days of absence, I am weary:
She I love is far away."
[JEAN-JACQUES ROUSSEAU — "Day of Absence"]

WHEN Mom was discharged from St. Joseph's in mid-November, the adjustment phase was no less difficult than with previous homecomings; 20 years of hospitalizations had set cruel precedents. Each time Mom came out of the hospital, it would take several days, if not weeks, to be sure she really was better. During those reintegration periods, it was always difficult to set aside the bitter arguing and struggling that routinely occurred during the extreme phases of her illness, and which could still flare up at any time. Every ounce of energy was required to focus on the matter at hand: shutting off the past and getting on with life.

That Mom rose in the morning before Dad went to work and us kids went off to school had always been a positive sign when Barry and I were growing up. Not until this happened for days running would we feel assured that the depression was at bay —at least for the time being. Yet deeply ingrained in us was the conditioned fear of relapse. We lived from remission to remission, ever bracing ourselves for the day when the buzzer on the kitchen stove would need to be reset over and over and over, signalling yet another downward spiral.

By that fall of 1982, our experience with Mom's recurring cycles of illness had so profoundly penetrated our lives that, despite the purported success of lithium, our confidence was in regrettably short supply. Mom's release from St. Joe's proved to be more of an anticlimax we embraced with a hardened and weathered wariness.

By the end of November 1982, Mom seemed to be relatively stable. When friends and relatives called, she would proudly inform them she was feeling much better. Everybody was relieved. Nobody could understand why, if lithium was working so well now, she couldn't have started taking it sooner.

At the time, Barry was immersed in his second year of Hospitality Services at George Brown College in Toronto. Dad was still employed as a draftsman at Bridge and Tank, and I was in the throes of my second year of French studies at McMaster University. With Mom back home, I felt the onus was on me to spend less time at the campus library in the evenings and more time around the house. For the first few days after her return, Mom, Dad, and I all tried to pick up where we had left off some six months prior, before the last episode of depression set in. That late fall was a period characterized by strain and uncertainty. With almost neurotic attention, I would be watching for the familiar signs that Mom was slipping; that the lithium was not working. It was simply too good to be true that after all those years something would finally set her free of depression. Nothing short of a miracle could have such a dramatic effect on our lives.

Night after night, when the dishes were done, I would forego the mounds of homework begging for my attention and spend time with Mom, both of us vacantly watching TV in the living room — hardly quality time. While Mom sat upright in the corner of the green upholstered couch with the gold-leaf patterns, I sat curled in the matching chair at the other side of the room. There we would remain for what seemed like hours, straining to make conversation during the too-frequent commercials, grateful for the return of some mundane program to fill the awkward silences. While Dad occupied himself downstairs or outside the house, I felt an enormous responsibility to fulfill Mom's need for the company of which she had been deprived for so long. In theory, those long evenings presented the perfect opportunity to share with her how relieved I was to have her home and "well." In an ideal world, it was a time to be happy, to celebrate. But sadness engulfed me, sitting with this woman, whom in the past I had actually feared at one time or another. I was at a loss as how to garner the happiness her presence now warranted.

And so I ate. I ate to counter the guilt of not being the daughter she needed to help ease her back into the family. I ate to fill the emptiness that consumed my body. At times, it was as if I was eating myself into a coma, distancing myself from my own inadequacy as her eldest offspring. In attempting to navigate the vast desert between us, I unwittingly constructed massive dunes of sand that provided insulation against those and other feelings. Regrettably, there were no fireworks to illuminate Mom's return from the shadow of death; only the bluish tinge of the television, accompanied by an inexplicable gloom that hovered overhead, and the unmistakable gnawing in my stomach that something was still not right.

(Summer 1994) It was one of those deathly still summer after-noons when my 93-year-old neighbour Impi phoned to ask if I could pop over to give her a hand. Knowing she had just had a new counter-top installed, I assumed she wanted me to help her put things back into the cupboards. When I arrived in her kitchen, I was taken aback. All of the cupboard doors were ajar, and on each of the shelves under the sink were huge chunks of Arborite and plaster, nesting in among all of her pots, pans, and cooking items, which had remained in place during the installation. The workmen had neglected to inform her to remove everything in advance, and certainly had not had the decency to do it themselves. While the new counter looked great, an elderly woman was left to contend with the debris.

As I proceeded to clean up the affected area, I was flooded with a wave of enlightenment; I flashed back to the fall of 1982, when Mom came home to begin her lithium life amidst the rubble of emotional debris. Ironically, though Dr. Reimer had "fixed" Mom with lithium, her depression had so long organized our lives that we were ill-prepared to handle the swelling tidal wave of wellness. Learning to cope without depression was unfamiliar; the predictable was now gone.

Clinical depression is an illness that impacts with often latent intensity on all members of a family. Yet through the years of Mom's cycles, there was never discussion, neither with professionals, nor amongst us as a family, about how Dad, Barry, and I were also affected. Neither was there guidance on how to support Mom in the way she most needed, both in sickness and in health. By 1982, we merely co-existed as strangers trapped under the same roof, as if inadvertently brought together by some quirk of fate. Much as the new psychiatrist was making headway with Mom (and Dad had even met him once or twice), there was still no concerted attempt to speak with Barry and me, or to the family together as a unit. Though four people's lives had all been intricately tangled together by two decades of depression, three of us were rendered nothing more than dislocated limbs of the person who was at the hub of it all. We were the walking wounded, and had unwittingly started spinning our own webs of false preservation.

Depression has somewhat of a teeter-totter effect on those who live with the afflicted individual. On the one hand, there is the pressure for significant others to be strong and supportive, to endure the illness and to just be there, often at the expense of their own feelings and emotions. On the other, living with a depressive is in itself depressing; it gets you down; it triggers a tendency to absorb the other's despondency. I have no doubt that my Dad, Barry, and I all fell prey to this phenomenon. In Dad's case, it was essentially a case of spousal see-saw syndrome.

Over the years, the responsibilities thrust upon him of home and work demanded Dad to be fully in control, often taking on the role of both parents, when Mom was in bed or hospitalized. In so doing, his needs took a back-seat for the better part of two decades. His life was no longer his own. With the exception of the curling club he belonged to in the 1970s, there was seldom respite from domestic and professional toils. That he never left our family as he so often threatened to do must initially have been out of a devotion to his wife and children. It later developed into a bitter martyrdom to tough it out, as the emotional distance between my parents grew out of the nightmare of Mom's recurring depression.

As a man who is known for his quick temper, Dad also bore the brunt of blame for his wife's cycles of depression. If the truth be known, there was no shortage of people who believed he "made" Mom that way. Ironically, I recall my Mom echoing her own mother's words that Dad's "bark is worse than his bite," as if that would somehow minimize the effect of his emotionally hurtful and psychologically damaging words. The years of explosive outbursts toward Mom as she lay helplessly in bed may well have been symptomatic of his internalized frustration. It takes an insightful and forgiving individual, however, to recognize that underneath Dad's hard exterior huddled someone who was hurting very much inside. For whatever baggage Dad brought into the marriage was left on the back burner when Mom had fallen ill barely four years after their 1958 honeymoon. The nurturing and acceptance he lacked in his own childhood had created an enormous well that he hungered to fill in adulthood. As a husband and father, I would venture he seldom came close to emotional fulfillment, what with a sick wife, two young children, and friends and family members who chastised him for being verbally abrasive with Mom. There was nobody there to fill his pitcher. Looking back, it is remarkable that Dad endured the strain of such a labour-intensive and socially isolating relationship. And the price he paid would be a high one.

Eighteen: Burning bridges

[MAY 8, 1985 — JOURNAL ENTRY] *Coming home 11:00 p.m. Dad really down. Looks awful; like he's ready to cry, but chokes out frustrated words instead. "Fed up with married life. Just feel like packing it in. Family, job — just sick of the whole goddamned life. Don't know what I'm gonna do. Maybe I'll just shoot myself . . ."*

BETWEEN THE years 1962 and 1982, Dad's emotional resistance to the vicious cycles of Mom's depression wore precariously thin, until there was a seamlessness between Mom's illness and his wellness — or vice versa. For when Mom improved, it was a silent nod to Dad that *"I'm okay now — you don't have to worry about me."* In short, the once-rigid roles and responsibilities become fuzzy, as Dad, the perennially caregiving mate of sorts, fell into a reactive depression.

In the months following Mom's release from hospital, however, these dynamics were not quite as apparent. In the spring of 1983, Dad decided that the house needed a change. For a one-income family, it was nothing less than a major overhaul. Over a period of several weeks, he and Mom went shopping together for new house trimmings. At the best of times, with the exception of grocery shopping, such mutual outings were virtual anomalies. Each of the three bedrooms and the dining room were dressed with custom-tailored drapes; the living room was adorned with full length honey-coloured ones as well as delicately pleated sheers, which made the house seem not nearly so dark. Ginger-brown wall-to-wall carpet throughout the living room and hallway was a welcome change from the well-worn teal that had been the ground cover for many a battle. A generously cushioned flowered sofa and matching chair, a copper-coloured Lazy-Boy, oak end- and coffee tables, along with new lamps, and the makeover was complete. However long Dad had been contemplating this cosmetic surgery, I could not help regarding it as symbolic of our family's new lease on life.

By December 1984, the lease expired, when the company my Dad had worked for as a draftsman over the past 38 years closed. It was a devastating experience to have the only livelihood he had known since the age of 16 ripped out from beneath him. At the time, I was struggling through my third year of university, and Barry was still living and studying in Toronto. Neither of us was able to offer the support he needed through that rough period. Growing up, Dad had rarely talked about his work — nor did we ask. We were never the share-your-day-over-dinner-type family. Regrettably, I was in my late 20s before I ever really looked at one of his blueprints and gained an appreciation for the complexity of the profession and the expertise it necessitated. When he was faced with the humbling experience of job-hunting at age 54, I had no frame of reference from which to help him, neither with the transition from stability to uncertainty, nor to soften the blow to his self-esteem when he accepted a position in early 1985, working under people many years his junior. If anybody, it was my Mom who became the emotional strength of the family. I shudder to think what would have happened if this shift had transpired in her pre-lithium era.

To this day, people still remark about how hard-hit Dad was about the company closure and that he has never been the same. A number of health problems, including inordinate fatigue, sleeplessness, and weight gain, may have masked a chronic level of depression within him; one that had been festering beneath the surface, as the spouse of a depressed woman, and fuelled by the job loss. He seemed to lapse into his own cocoon of emotional neediness, a desperate lament for years of unrealized hopes and dreams. For to his tremendous credit, my Dad stayed in a situation that many men would have left years prior. Throughout all the years he invested taking care of the family, the dividends were negligible. There was no nurturing husband–wife relationship to relish or a blossoming father–daughter bond to take solace in when the lithium stock was offered as payback.

[MAY 8, 1985 — JOURNAL ENTRY] *Mom and I are both frozen in place in the dining room, Dad now sitting in the kitchen with his head in his hands. I'm scared for Dad, for Mom; what does life hold for them? Togetherness suddenly seems unlikely, though separate is equally unfathomable. I'm scared to go to sleep. What if Dad does something to all of us? Call Barry ...*

In the spring of 1985, when Dad began stagnating in his own depression, Dr. MacIntosh told him he had no reason to be down in the dumps. "You've already been through this with your wife for 20 years. Shake yourself out of it," I once heard Dad tell someone of the good doctor who had chided him. One thing about Dr. MacIntosh: he remained pathetically consistent with his remedies for depression. All he did was cough up the same useless rhetoric he'd preached to Mom for those same 20 years. Hippocratic oath be damned. Where were his warmth, sympathy, and understanding? What about caring for others, as he would have them care for him?

Though my parental allegiance had always been with my mom, I couldn't help but think of how living through two decades of his wife's depression virtually entitled my Dad to be depressed.

[MAY 9, 1985 — JOURNAL ENTRY] *Dad still down, just sitting in his chair in the living room with a second pot of tea. If anyone calls, he's sleeping. Whispers to me when he passes that it's his nerves. "I'll tell you later," he says, meaning after Mom leaves for her group meeting, and knowing that I have a day off. What will I do if he breaks down, I wonder. How it pains me to see him so sad looking, his face lined, mouth drawn down around the corners, hurt in his eyes, like a puppy dog. He is such a great man, and he probably doesn't even know I think that way. When have I ever told him that I love him? Never. But then I have never been able to tell Mom either, the two people who need to hear it the most. Want so much to hug him, to apologize for the daughter I am. I could be more of a companion, but it is hard — I do try as often as I can, but it's just he's so moody and I am so afraid of being criticized that I just come and go pretty much. But I'm moody too — my own problems that get me down and living at home just makes matters worse — though it's not really them, it's me. When have I thanked him for sticking around all those years, going through hell, more out of obligation than love? I could always run to friends, get away, no matter how obligated I felt to stay here. What made me think I was so entitled that way while Dad stuck around? My obligation was as great as his; perhaps it could be argued ever greater, because I am her flesh and blood, whereas they are just joined by marriage . . .*

"Later" came all too soon that day. I had barely finished writing those words when Dad came into my room. It was 10:00 a.m. on a beautiful spring morning, which swiftly clouded with Dad's confession that he had "met someone." Blood had drained from my face before, but never quite like that. "It's nothing sexual," he was quick to assure me, as if that made it okay. I was weak, but managed to stand, numbed and trapped by this speech I certainly did not ask to hear. He continued, oblivious to the effect his purge was having on me — his daughter, not his psychiatrist.

"There is no love between your mother and me — that stopped six or seven years ago," he explained. Going on about how he enjoys the company of this woman; she's not like the others he has met. As if he had not antagonized my parents' acrimonious relationship enough over the years, Dad's primary defense for his indiscretion was that Dr. MacIntosh encouraged him to go ahead — he sees it every day and people in worse situations than Dad and Mom have gone through things okay.

I was seething inside. How could he do this to Mom now? Yet somehow, I heard myself telling Dad that I could understand how he would do something like that, thinking it had probably kept him alive, gave him a reason to live. Whether or not he took that as my blessing for his continued trysts, he kept talking, explaining how it had happened, what a good friend she was, how lonely he had been. But I was already tuned out. When he sensed I didn't want to hear anymore, the tables turned. Suddenly, he challenged me about why I didn't have a boyfriend. What the hell that had to do with his infidelity was beyond me. My retort was a snappy "I don't have a very good example of relationships, do I?" Momentarily, I regretted my tone, wondering what he was leading to. None too soon, he left my room, slamming the door behind him. I felt sick and ashamed of myself for letting him invade my life like that, dumping his problems in my lap. How was I to face him anymore? Or, more importantly, how could I face Mom? For this knowledge put me in a position of betrayal; an unwilling co-conspirator to my Dad's unfaithfulness.

Dad's disclosure should have come as no surprise, for I had long harboured suspicions about why he always spent so much time "at the butcher shop" on Friday nights. Certainly it was something that could have manifested itself years earlier, as their marriage was ripped apart by Mom's depression. I had always worried what would happen to my parents when Barry and I got older. That day, I was taken off guard. It flashed through my mind Dad was finally going to leave, and that I would have to forfeit my final year of university and subsequent plans to travel abroad, so that I could find a job to support Mom. After more than two years stabilized on lithium, now this. How on earth would Mom be able to handle such a breach of trust? I was sickened with Dad's imposition on me. I couldn't figure out why he was telling me. In retaliation, I invited a couple of friends over and proceeded to get progressively drunk in my own backyard. The evening sun had barely set when I passed out for the night. Life always seemed to present reasons to run.

[May 20, 1985 — journal entry] *Dad still really bummed out — has been two solid weeks now; six weeks off and on altogether. Mom tries to reassure me, says he'll be okay — "it's just one of those things — not very nice," and attributes his mood to problems at his new job. I can't handle it. If he's not sitting and staring vacantly out the window, he's moping somewhere else — on the stairs with head in his hands — so listless I can't face him. After so many years with Mom being down, same thing all over, yet somehow scarier, because Dad is supposed to be so bloody strong.*

The day finally came when Mom asked if I knew about Dad's "friend." She was sitting on the edge of her bed with dry tears in her eyes. I was shaking, certain this was the setback we had all feared. I was also afraid she'd think the whole thing was a conspiracy against her. I walked over to her and gave her the biggest hug I could, telling her how guilty I had felt ever since I'd known. Despite the bitterness of betrayal, that day bore witness to the stabilizing effect of lithium. Mom was okay. And I had the burden of keeping Dad's secret lifted from my shoulders. From that day forward, yet another elephant joined the herd standing in the living room that was never again to be discussed.

Light years before Dad's first warning signs of cracking, I'd slipped into my own altered state. I was insulated by the comfort of substance versus love. During the transition from my teens into my twenties, for every time Dad lamented how he was "so screwed up" and didn't know how to think or feel anymore, I screamed inside, wanting to rip out my guts and throw them down at his feet. What the hell did he think I was going through? Did he not wonder why I had been coming home drunk since the age of fifteen? Never once did he ask me how on earth I was managing everything in my life. After years of the world revolving around Mom, I detested the fact that now everything was about him. How angrily I swallowed the bitter bile of a retort festering within when he lapsed so pathetically into his "woe is me" dramatics, moping around the house demanding pity and compassion. The whole of me was dying to shout back, "I don't give a fuckin' shit about you! What about me?" But there was no room for such dramatics, or such honesty. In that household, as far as I was, and remain, concerned, there never had been, and never would be, any constructive outlet for all the years of smothered fear and anger, born of my mother's depression and of bearing witness to my parents' bitter physical and emotional fighting. Whatever childhood and teenage problems and difficulties I may have been forced to contend with had long been better left unsaid. And there my formative years would remain, trapped inside with no verbal means of escape, for the bridges of communication between all of us, and most definitely between my Dad and me, had long ago been burned.

Nineteen: Disordered daughter

[DECEMBER 1982] *Litre of rainbow sherbet nestled in lap. TV program about female inmates in the Kingston Prison for Women. Disturbing accounts of self-mutilation. Time passes. Growing sense of unease. Spooning way to bottom of container. Reality gels. Panic. Waves of nausea descend. Paralyzed with fear. Oh my God. What have I done? Lift self from couch. Robotically make way to bathroom. Exhausted. Alone. Afraid. Cry self to sleep ...*

When Mom was released from St. Joseph's Hospital in November 1982, it was also as if it was a nod, not unlike the one directed at Dad, for me to start focusing on myself: Mom was "okay." I must have misinterpreted that toss of the medicine ball, however, as it was almost like clockwork that the wick of my internal time bomb, ignited at 16, flared up with a fervor. Twenty years out of the womb, I was an explosion waiting to happen.

Faced with mid-term exams, Mom's homecoming, weight gain, and general emotional upheaval, I made a difficult decision to temporarily move out of my parents' home. All I needed was a place to sleep and study for a month. Initially, the downtown YWCA, where I had taken swimming lessons for years as a child, offered a familiarity and was the only reasonably priced place that came to mind. But as luck would have it, my friend Wendy offered the use of her apartment, as she was seldom there. Much as I felt I was deserting my parents during their time of need, I was pulled toward a faint voice of self-preservation in order to salvage my studies. So at the beginning of December 1982, with the help of my brother, who was home for a weekend, I moved books, clothes, records, and a few personal items into Wendy's apartment on Forest Avenue, mere blocks from St. Joseph's Hospital, from where Mom had recently been released. Not so coincidentally, my temporary home was in the part of the city just below the Hamilton escarpment, and near the stairway leading to the Ontario Psychiatric Hospital, where Mom had first been hospitalized in December 1962.

For the first time in my life, I answered only to myself. The aloneness was disconcerting at first, but I soon adopted a routine of classes, studying, working two part-time jobs and coming back to the apartment to sleep. Things were going well. I began losing weight, primarily because there was no food in the fridge. One night, returning from school, I came to a halt outside the local IGA store on James Street South, overwhelmed with the need to reward myself for the weight I had lost so far. Wandering inside, I made my way to the frozen food section, where it was a container of rainbow sherbet that lured me. Calorie-wise, not as bad as ice cream, I assured myself as I paid for my purchase and walked the couple of blocks to the apartment.

I settled myself on the couch and proceeded to eat straight from the container. Having had nothing all day save for numerous cups of coffee, I told myself I was legitimately hungry. But the other part of my brain knew better: it was more than physical hunger. It was as if I was eating to fill an emotional and psychological void; that of being alone and trying to deal with the guilt of abandoning Mom. There was also the stress of exams and papers, on top of the ever-present sexual identity conflict within. A myriad of thoughts vied for time in my brain, and before I knew it, I had devoured the entire container. What had begun innocently enough proved to be quite the opposite. I had lost the control I had fought to regain over the previous couple of weeks. I panicked. Whether I legitimately felt sick or I couldn't bear the thought of having eaten so much, I cannot be certain. What was certain was that the initial upheaval catapulted me further along the road of self-destruction. How different was I than those incarcerated women in Kingston's "P4W," who thrived on the tattooed markings of their own carved and shredded skin? The flesh of my soul seemed to crave the same pain.

I lay in bed that night, frozen by fear of the unknown, trying to block out random thoughts of the unspeakable deed. And I awoke the next morning afraid of the day. All hopes that the incident was an isolated occurrence were cruelly dashed when "it" happened again a few days later ... and again ... and again ... and again. By the time I went home to my parents for Christmas, I had lost 15 pounds and gained an eating disorder. I felt good about my weight loss, but distressed about the method and the pattern that was emerging. Still, I rationalized that it would stop because I had almost met my weight-loss goal, and the pressure of exams was over.

Back in my parents' home, I was even more of a stranger than when I had left three weeks prior, for the cycle of bingeing, purging, and starving had taken a grip on my life in a way that was quickly proving to be more encompassing and relentless than that of alcohol. Riddled with shame about what I was doing, I further isolated myself. I was no longer myself. I was a full-blown bulimic.

The sound of Christmas carols around our house has always been about as popular as that of nails on a chalkboard, making you want to shout, "STOP!" Christmas Day had always been a judgment day of sorts: would Mom make it? That first lithium Christmas in 1982, Mom was fine. But the trumpets were silent, genuine happiness eluded us, like a buried treasure beneath the snow that blanketed our house on the hill. I was like the traditional tin soldier, rigid and unfeeling in my emotions toward my family, wanting only to ride away from it all, into some distant never-never land.

On the threshold of 1983, in light of Mom's continued wellness, we had every reason to be popping the champagne and welcoming the

New Year: out with the old and in with the new indeed. As for my resolutions to stop the bingeing and purging, they fell quickly by the wayside. What I thought may have been uncharted territory, had in fact been carefully navigated since Barry and I began throwing away morsels of food we did not like or could not finish when we were young. From that point on, erratic eating patterns during high school had been commonplace, as food became the enemy and wielded a powerful influence over my shaky teenage self-esteem. Bulimia was almost the next logical phase of a pre-existing struggle with substance abuse and emotions. After so many years of restrictive eating and guilty indulgences, I had gone past the point of no return.

Eventually, the eating disorder was all consuming, distancing me from the world, and enveloping me in a shroud of perpetual fear. At a time when Mom needed me the most to support her continued state of health, I was drifting further away. On the surface, it made no sense to anyone why I was so down when the most significant worry in my life was remedied. It was as if the longer Mom stayed better, I had permission to focus on the issues and feelings so long suppressed. In doing so, the pressure cooker of internalized emotion exploded. I proceeded to crumble into smaller and smaller pieces until there was but a scattered heap of rubble from which to reconstruct myself years later. Though I could no longer hide from myself, at all cost, I had to smother my feelings and hide from others. It was clear that alcohol was no longer enough: I needed a more accessible and socially accept-able substance.

Just as I'd been drinking since high school to escape from Mom's depression, my parents arguing, and my internal struggles about Mrs. Michaels, so eating offered a means of escape — from the new dynamics of Mom's wellness, and from the self it was becoming more difficult to avoid. Food served me well by suffocating thoughts, feel-ings, and inadequacies I could not control. It was like cutting off the air supply to my very essence. Yet the need to repress my inner self was paramount, for fear that if my parents ever found out my true nature, it would cause Mom to relapse. For so many years, I had tried to be a strong and dutiful daughter. Then, as my own issues and emotions came into the fore, I perceived myself as a fraud: a terrible daughter, sister, friend, co-worker, and person. Shielding the outside world from knowing me, I almost killed myself in the process. At the best of times, I was depressed and aloof, frightened of the way the eating disorder had taken control of me. Destructive eating and drinking went hand in hand. Purging, then soothing the roughness of my throat with cold beer or warm whiskey, became a pattern I despised yet embraced.

[FEBRUARY 1983] Determined to put an end to the bulimia once and for all, I made an appointment with Dr. Ted Jones, a lanky and bored-looking psychiatrist to whom I'd been referred by a friend who had dated his son. When I explained what had brought me to see him, I wished I'd never walked through the door. He trivialized the eating patterns I knew were clearly unhealthy, sarcastically asking, "What do you eat, a couple of crackers — maybe with peanut butter — then go make yourself throw it up?" I was humiliated beyond words. I could think of nothing to offer in response before he brazenly asked me if there was a connection between eating and sex. I froze. How could he possibly know? I had long fought to ignore the pressure cooker on the back burner since I first noticed the lid lifting at the tender age of five. In my teens, I began clamping it down with alcohol. In my twenties, the alcohol did not suffice. To a degree, I had come to associate the bingeing and purging as another way to suppress my sexual self. My homosexuality. Now, it felt as if it was being thrown in my face by some dinosaur of a psychiatrist whose manner was not in the least conducive to disclosure. I vehemently denied it, knowing I had to get out of there as soon as possible. The remainder of the session was a blur. I vowed never again to discuss my eating problem — let alone my sexuality — with another shrink, certainly not a male one.

By March 1983, I weighed 103 pounds. I was thrilled. But I was also anxious, for I didn't know how I would manage a two-week vacation down to Florida with my friend Leanne, her mother, and her younger sister, Lisa. We would be staying at her grandparents' summer home, in a retirement village near Fort Myers. I had not been to Florida since I was five, so I was looking forward to visiting as an adult. However, bingeing and purging was an almost daily ritual by then, and I was not at all certain how I could manage being in such close quarters with people.

As it turned out, those fourteen days proved to be the longest stretch of "remission" I would have for the next five years. I was so caught up in the carefreeness of the holiday that spending time with Leanne and her easy-going family was truly restorative. Though I had known Leanne for only about two-and-a-half years, her home in Hamilton had often been an oasis for me during times of emotional drought. She and her mother, Elaine, made sure I knew their door was always open. Those two weeks were precious respite from myself, as I indulged myself in their laughter and love.

For the next year and a half, my eating disorder progressed to a magnitude beyond my greatest fears. Though I did tentatively broach my concerns with two friends, Jenny and Susan, I conveniently masked the severity, such that neither they, nor I, ever brought it up again. As the bulimia escalated, I continued to be haunted by Dr. Jones' pointed question. It was too close for comfort. Much as I still tried to deny it, the issue was boldly clawing its way to the surface, begging for attention. What was I so afraid of that I needed alcohol and food to buffer my burgeoning sexuality? I could conjure up a host of worst-case scenarios: friends would leave; Dad would be furious;

Barry would be disgusted. By far the greatest fear was that it would trigger Mom's relapse. Though I'd never been able to control Dad's anger or Mom's depression, I'd worked too long and too hard to keep them at bay to drop this nuclear bomb in their midst. It was safer to remain an island unto myself.

Canadian singer-songwriter Jane Siberry's mournfully melodic voice resonated within during a concert at Toronto's Massey Hall in the mid 1980s. My eyes welled up, as if she were singing her moving ballad "You Don't Need" directly to me. Though I was present in the physical sense in my day-to-day life, I was unreachable, all but alienating even my closest of friends, to whom I could not confide how sick and confused I was.

[MARCH 1984] A trip to Quebec City with my friend Susan and the French Club at McMaster University was, at the time, the pinnacle of angst for me. As departure day loomed, I was increasingly despondent and all consumed by the wrath of bulimia. Social situations at best were difficult, not to mention spending several days surrounded by a busload of people. With only days to spare, I told Susan I did not feel up to going. Understandably, she was upset, particularly when I could not fully express how I was feeling. After all, everybody gets down.

Unable to shoulder the guilt of backing out at the last minute, I ended up going for the sake of our friendship. From the time I boarded the bus until the time I came home, I drank. Peppermint schnapps, vodka and orange juice, beer, and the wonderfully traditional Winter Carnival beverage "Caribou," a potent mixture of red wine and straight alcohol. To others who knew me as an unassuming member of the French Club, I came across as a shy, yet willing partier. But beneath the surface, I was screaming for solitude. When I could, I escaped from the evening's gatherings to the sanctity of my hotel room, or out to the streets of the Old City, the glow of alcohol a comfort against the bitter cold Quebec night. By day, crossing The Plains of Abraham, I ached to leave my battle-weary body behind for the winds off the St. Lawrence to whip over for the rest of eternity.

Had it not been for a friend named Mimi, I could have lost myself in the Hades of bulimia without a soul ever knowing. She was the only person at that time that I allowed to drift close when the waves of nothingness came crashing upon my shore. We communicated even when there was silence on the other end of the telephone line, or across the café table where we'd meet for a drink. Though I never divulged my innermost struggle of sexuality until years later, there was an unspoken acceptance and understanding of my desperate battle with food. For the dark hell of an eating disorder can be shared only by one who has tasted the bitter self-destructiveness as it heaves within over and over and over.

Though my shame and pride prevented me from confiding in her at times when I most needed to, she was only a call away when, my throat still raw and the tears carving salt-stained rivers upon my face, I would phone, just to hear her comforting voice. For a number of years, she did more for me than any psychiatrist or counsellor. Though the sands of time were scorching beneath my feet, the wave of her friendship rolled up and cooled me, and kept me from drowning off the coast of my deserted island in the black sea of despondency. Ironically, though I had lived through 20 years of Mom's depression, I did not know to how handle my own despair. Neither did I reach out to her — my own Mother — as a source of support, despite her wealth of "expertise." I had too much to tell and too little courage. I chose instead isolation from the very woman who gave me birth, virtually eating, fasting, and drinking my way toward the great leveller — the great escape.

Twenty: Meeting the mountain

[AUGUST 1984 — JOURNAL ENTRY] *"What the hell are you doing?" I yell at myself. No answer of course. I cannot understand the grip of this compulsion at all . . .*

IN THE SUMMER of 1984, a twist of fate turned the tables in my favour. Unable to sleep after my nightshift summer job at the university, I happened to turn on the television — something I was not in the habit of doing mid-day. Flicking the channels as I ate my way through a box of Ritz-like crackers, I stopped at the local *Cherrington* phone-in talk show. A private counsellor by the name of Dianna Drummond was talking about her work with sufferers of eating disorders. I felt the blood drain from my face as it does when there is instantaneous connection with something unpleasant.

At the end of the program, I took down her mailing address and resolved to contact her in Toronto. I put as much as I felt necessary to convey in the letter, hesitating not to reveal my deep, dark secret of bulimia to this virtual stranger. Several weeks later, I received a most compassionate letter of response from her. She acknowledged how all-consuming an eating disorder can be and praised the courage she knew it had taken to share my story with her. Yet where she saw courage, I felt only weakness and shame, for I had reached out to her in desperation. Her correspondence conveyed an uncanny belief in me, someone she had met but through a single letter. It was almost unsettling. Her message to me was one of hope; her words embraced me as warmly as a tightly woven blanket through a never-ending winter. "Please take care of you now," she wrote, "it is your turn."

Dianna offered to take me on as a client, and the 25 dollars a week in addition to the return bus fare to Toronto gave me hope that things would finally change for the better. My counselling sessions with her provided respite from the wrath of myself — if only for a few hours. I found solace in the two-hour hike from the bus terminal up to her home-office, north of Avenue Road and Eglinton Avenue; a long but necessary journey I'd make by foot. I allowed myself to be drawn into the serenity of Dianna's surroundings, feeling somehow at home with this woman my mother's age, in a way I had never been in my parents' house. But that was more about Dianna than it was about me. Her pitcher of goodness was overflowing; I the bearer of an emotional well, long run dry. Her essence was spiritual, and I a lost soul at her mercy, desperate for healing.

As Dianna slowly and quietly inhaled her cigarette, her eyes would squint closed ever so slightly as she gazed at me more intently than anyone ever had since Mrs. Michaels back in high school. It was during those moments that I felt she was inside me. She told me things about myself I had never wanted to know and was reluctant to believe. She gently but firmly encouraged me to talk of my feelings, fears, anxieties, and emotions instead of using food to cope with them. At the end of each session, as I readied myself to depart, Dianna would hug me tightly as if to infuse in me the necessary belief in self I would need to carry me through the days so darkened without her light. It was not lost on me how different it felt for me to be in Dianna's presence than with my own mother; certainly the "therapeutic" hugs she provided were stronger, firmer, and longer lasting than any I had ever shared with my own mother.

The time until the next session with her was endless for me. Beyond the security of her presence and positive affirmations, I was alone in my private hell back in Hamilton. Try as I might, I was light-years away from acquiring the peace of mind and self-nurturing she counselled was paramount to recovery.

Between sessions, Dianna suggested I contact a woman named Pam, who was then working at one of the McMaster libraries. "Pam is a very unique and remarkable person. Find her, Nancy. She will welcome you with open arms and will guide you on your way. She is well and whole because she wanted it. I feel you do too." The day I sought Pam out in mid-September 1984, I was a bundle of nerves, try-ing to appear as nonchalant as possible as I hovered around the department where she worked. Of the two women there, I had the frail and rather pale-looking one pegged as the Pam I was seeking. Waiting until I saw her leave, I nervously approached the other woman and asked for Pam. When she introduced herself as Pam, I was caught off guard, for I was unprepared for such a sudden meeting. Nevertheless, my words came fumbling out. Fortunately, Dianna had spoken of me to Pam, and I did not have to say much. Her vibrant and earthy nature instantly appealed to me. Over the next few weeks, we established a friendship that will endure a lifetime. She was an energy that electrified my private hell.

Soon we organized an informal support group, which at times included my friend Mimi and another woman, Winnie. We were four souls drifting, yet clinging to the preservers we threw out to each other. Much as I may have been able to share aspects of my eating disorder, my family, my feelings of depression, and general life anxi-ety, it was everything that was left unsaid that kept me from getting "better." Though the connection between bulimia and my sexuality was paramount in my mind, it was a piece of the puzzle I remained committed to sharing with nobody, not even Mimi or Pam, who showed every sign of accepting me unconditionally. I remained scared as hell to admit my sexuality to another living soul, let alone to myself. At times, I was even too tired to keep writing about it, so I taped a series of messages, further punishing myself by later listening to the sound of my pathetic voice.

From time to time, occasionally when on the brink of a binge, though usually not until the deed done, I battled myself to remain still long enough to listen to a relaxation tape from Dianna. Her soft and rich melodic voice seeped through my ears and called upon my imagination. She invited me to visualize a favourite spot in nature, perhaps where the birds were in song, the breeze was gentle, the sky was blue, the sun was warm, and a stream was flowing. She beckoned me down a forested path, where, ahead in the distance, I would come upon a friendly face whose twinkling eyes would draw me into the light of life and out of the consuming darkness of daily living. I hungered to be bathed in the light, to be enveloped by the peace of mind that she suggested merely needed to be found after so long being covered up or forgotten. How was I to locate something I had no memory of ever having? Peace of mind was but a wishful state of being that belonged to someone else. As Dianna's voice reminded me, peace of mind cannot be achieved without making peace with the body. But I was at war on both mind and body fronts. As long as I held tight to the crutch of bulimia, my body was enslaved to my mind. Discard the crutch and peel off the mask, for what price need be paid to avoid reality and keep the world away?

Dianna's affirmations about the miracle of life and the joy of the child within were jaded by the abject negativity of my existence. I conceded only that it was a miracle I was still alive, given the way I treated my body. As for childhood and joy, they were not equated in my mind. I could not visualize myself on the screen of my life as anything other than a hollow mass of flabby skin, clinging to a mask carved with non-sparkling eyes and forced smiles — quite unlike the picture of myself the tape encouraged me to paint. How sparkling my eyes and radiant my smile could be if only I would lay down the burden of struggling with my soul, of remaining hostage to very human emotions, thoughts, and feelings. "Say what you have been dying to say," her recorded voice implored. How I wished I could release all the guilt, shame, fear, and sadness within me. The only expressions allowed were sobs of despair and binge after binge. I prayed for the willpower to transcend the bondage of bulimia, but somehow did not feel I deserved to be set free; it was a penance of sorts to suffer. Though I recognized the need for dramatic change, there was far too much inside of me that remained to be purged.

[OCTOBER 1984 — TAPED MESSAGE] *Dear God, please give me the strength to stop this shit. I just can't take it anymore. Feel frenzied, as if some demon possessing me to do it. Feel so alone …*

Two years after the onset of my eating disorder, I could no longer dismiss the physical implications of what the constant purging was doing to my body. On the recommendation of Dianna, I finally dredged up the nerve to speak with a nurse at the university student clinic. A kindly woman with a comforting manner, she spoke with me at length about the damage I was most likely doing to my body. She also expressed concern over my emotional and mental health. Despite my reluctance, she referred me to a "doctor" at the McMaster Medical Centre. When I made my way across campus to the appointment a few days later, a bitter November wind whipped through my facade of courage, my heart pounding with anxiety. When I arrived at the fourth-floor wing where the doctor's office was located, I stopped cold when I read the tiny letters on the wall: "Psychiatry." It somehow had not registered that I would be seeing a psychiatrist. Memories of Mom's psychiatrists and my brief encounter with Dr. Jones the year previous flooded my head. Before I could turn and run, a voice was asking my name. Caught, I could do nothing more than choke out who I was, and follow the receptionist's curt nod toward a pink vinyl seat. I sat and I waited, feeling immensely self-conscious all the while. How on earth did I end up here — the only psychiatric ward in the city in which Mom hadn't been confined. How was I to rid myself of the awful notion that I was breaking frightening new ground?

[NOVEMBER 1984 — TAPED MESSAGE] *Feel myself on the brink of going nuts. No control is the scariest thing I can imagine. Most lonely and frightening time of my life. Need to get away. Comfort and security of home is bullshit. I'm frightened to be here . . .*

For three months, I had weekly sessions with a diminutive psychiatric social worker named Linda, whose pursed lips and clinical questions did little to put me at ease as she herself sat perfectly rigid in her chair across from me. Though it must have had somewhat of a cathartic effect to talk about my depression, eating problem, and other aspects of my life, I was not very cooperative when it came down to the nitty-gritty about what was bothering me. The sizeable diamond ring with accompanying wedding band, and the photos of her kids staring at me from her desk, did nothing to assure me this woman could understand the crux of my turmoil. I also was not entirely convinced there was nobody observing me behind the two-way mirror on one wall of the room, a common fixture in teaching hospitals such as McMaster — particularly on the psychiatric wards. Week after week, I dreaded Linda's patronizing stares and ruthless inquisitions. I felt trapped in a world I no longer wanted to be in...

I fantasized about forfeiting this anxiety along with my worldly possession, and taking refuge in the serenity of the Hare Krishna Temple I'd recently visited in Toronto in conjunction with a religious studies class I was taking. The allure of embracing a near monastic life, paying homage to a deity I knew only little about, was an enticing way to take shelter from the devilish forces inside me. Safe within a rigidly structured world was the only way I could think of to gain control of my life. I was stopped short of donning a flowing burnt-orange robe, shaving my head, and hawking incense by the tearful concern of my rational-minded friend Sharon, and long conversations with another friend Trisha, both who knew me enough to be alarmed by my despondent vulnerability. I relented, and tolerated Linda until February, when she left her interim position with McMaster to return to her full-time one with the Hamilton Psychiatric Hospital. I was then given the option of continuing the counselling with another "doctor."

[DECEMBER 1984 — TAPED MESSAGE] *Falling, falling down this cliff. Can't seem to grab on to anything. Just this shovel and it's digging me deeper and deeper . . .*

Though I was somewhat relieved I wouldn't have to endure more sessions with Linda, I did not warm to the thought of starting from square one with someone else. My rational brain told me that the eating disorder was so far out of control that I had no choice but to continue. And so I was assigned a resident in psychiatry named Morgan. Although the concept of therapy still made me nervous and anxious, Morgan had a captivating presence, which put me more at ease than I had been with her predecessor. Her approach was more intense, in that she seldom asked questions, waiting until I spoke first. Her eyes bore through me in a way that subtly challenged me to connect with her, stirring up feelings that had taken root back in high school English class with Mrs. Michaels. It drove me nuts. It often compelled me to eat and purge right up until the time I had to leave for a session. How many times did I arrive with puffy eyes and broken blood vessels upon my cheeks, my throat so parched I could barely talk, silently beseeching her to see how serious my problem was? Though I still beat around the bush and thrashed about in the closet for months, the dynamics with her were different, and I could feel myself shifting slightly toward a less hostile view of therapy. But my thoughts were ridden with personal abasement: my self-esteem tattered; my body image distorted; my life a cyclical purge in the name of escape.

[MAY 1985 — JOURNAL ENTRY] *Am very desperate to have them done. As small as possible — flat even, I don't care. Just do it. If I could cut them off, I would . . .*

"It" was a reduction mammoplasty. That there was a medical term for breast reducing somehow justified my emotional and psychological need to undergo such a procedure. By the standards of the few friends who knew what I wanted to do, it was an extreme measure to fool with Mother Nature in such a fashion. But Mother Nature had already dealt me a heavy blow at birth, by whisking my own mother away; I believed I had nothing to lose by shrinking the space I took up in the world. Though I never consciously perceived it to be so at the time, the obsession to alter my body in such a radical way has since been challenged by professionals and friends alike as being an extension of my self-destructive tendency. But I hid behind the physical reasoning: the shoulder gouges and chest abrasions that are inevitable when a large-breasted woman runs miles a day with a heavy underwire bra.

I spoke with Morgan at length about my desire for the surgery, and the effect it would have on my life. Never once did she challenge my motive or rationale. In hindsight, the disgust with my body, and pervasive self-loathing, was all-consuming, and I would have paid little heed to anyone who tried to stop me — even Morgan. That was saying a lot, as at that time, Morgan was probably the only person I trusted enough to provide me with desperately needed objectivity. Surgery was a way to have control over something in my life; to become less noticeable in a world in which I was becoming dangerously confused and scared to find myself in. The risk of complications — or disfigurement — did not even enter into the equation as a factor to consider. Neither did a caution from a close friend about her experience with the same surgeon's sexual impropriety when she underwent an operation with him a couple of years prior. And indeed he did cross the line of professionalism on more than one occasion with me: commenting on the "beauty" of my breasts and massaging my shoulders during the initial consultation meeting; massaging my pelvic area during the post-surgical follow-up when the stitches were to be removed. On both occasions, he suggested I call him any time, should I need help adjusting to my new breasts. Disgusted as I was, he was a means to an end for me. The deed was done. Weeks of post-operative pain were a small price to pay for how much freer I felt in my body.

On the grand scheme of things, I was lucky. Three years later, in February 1988, when he was brought up before the College of Physicians and Surgeons on charges of professional misconduct for sexually assaulting two young girls, the son-of-a-bitch committed suicide. I was shaken when I read about it in the *Hamilton Spectator*. I clipped the article, reading it over and over as I drank myself into a stupor: had I passively condoned his wrongful behaviour — perhaps at the expense of younger and more vulnerable patients? I can only console myself, years later, in knowing I was hardly in a position of emotional stability to have taken the necessary steps to address his blatant infractions of the revered Hippocratic oath. Worse than his legacy I carry forever upon my chest, is the deep-seated mistrust I have about medical professionals. Anyone worth their weight in gold needs to win my trust and confidence more than is measurable.

[JUNE 1985 — JOURNAL ENTRY] *Exhausted mess as usual. Can't trust myself to feel good. Dad is pissing me off. There is no talking to him rationally. Mom has come so far, but he is still so goddamned demeaning. He talks to her like shit. There is no way she should have to tolerate that kind of language. Really gets me down ...*

In the post-operative summer of 1985, on the verge of my final year of university, I took flight from my parents' home, primarily in an attempt to escape the uncomfortable triangle that had evolved with the knowledge of my Dad's infidelity, and his unrelenting emotional wearing down of Mom and me. Logistically, it may not have made sense to live away from home in the same city while still in school. I also had to deal with the guilt of again abandoning Mom. But the guilt excuse did not hold much water with many friends, notably Elaine and Pam, who cautioned that I didn't want to be one of those unmarried women getting into the rut of caring for their mother without ever having lived for themselves. Besides, Mom had been depression-free for nearly three years, during which time I had been a less than communicative daughter. Perhaps leaving would be for the better. I forged ahead with my decision. In a turn-of-the-century brownstone walkup with high ceilings and wooden floors on Duke Street, in one of my favourite parts of the city, I was nearer to a sense of self than I had ever been. The first evening I allowed myself to sit down with a book, Shirley MacLean's *Out on a Limb*, baroque music filling the room, candles and incense to calm. I cried, for the taste of such peace was a foreign one.

Living alone in the past had been a nightmare; I feared I was setting myself up for more serious alcohol and food problems. Though the bulimia did not fully remit and my drinking remained heavy, I felt liberated from the confines of being a dutiful daughter. Ultimately, as I gravitated toward more independence and a sense of self, the sessions with Morgan seemed to keep pointing in one direction. Week after week, I would hope to have the guts to disclose my deep dark secret. Week after week, we would sit there and stare at each other — or more so she at me as I focused on the world outside her window. Her silence was crazy-making for me, as I'm sure my frustrating silences were for her.

[November 1985 — journal entry] *I care about my family and friends so much, but they don't even fucking know me. Nobody does. How long can I go on . . .*

Since discussing an issue with Morgan as personal in nature as my operation earlier in the summer, I'd found myself slowly hedging toward a place I was not sure I would be comfortable. But something about the way she interacted with me started leading me out of my clouded existence. In November 1985, I released the enormous weight of sexual orientation from my significantly reduced chest. In the small, windowless room we were relegated to for that session, and with a disproportionate degree of intensity of my own creation, I divulged what I had been circling around for months. *I'm gay.* As soon as the words were out of my mouth, I was dizzy with fear, shame, and, strangely, relief. I was sure I could never bring myself to go back and see her. But I did. And it was paradoxically easier to sit across from her and talk, even though what I had disclosed to her relegated me to a vulnerable place with which I was not at all familiar.

Over the months of working with Morgan, I had gradually started to develop a trust in her, and a sense that maybe she could relate to me more than she was at liberty to reveal. I was therefore crestfallen when Morgan informed me in December that she was leaving; she was going off on another internship rotation. I was deeply saddened and experienced a sense of loss that was difficult to conquer. I was once again alone with my secret.

The unburdening with Morgan had nevertheless been a turning point. The New Year looked more promising than any one in recent memory. Five months later, by the grace of a force beyond me, I made it to my university graduation: May 31, 1986. Arriving at 6:30 a.m. on the campus to pick up my gown that May day, a slight hangover prevailed. Inconsequential. I had made it. After five long years, an Honours Bachelor of Arts Degree in French was mine. *Incroyable, mais vrais. Incredible, but true.* Act Two was over.

Twenty-one: Touching clouds

"Eventually, he hid himself away, on the heights of Mount Pilatus, and dwelt alone among the clouds and crags for years ...

[MARK TWAIN — *A Tramp Abroad*]

WITH BOTH tremendous relief and apprehension, in August 1986, I set off with a rucksack and a sleeping bag on a year-long sabbatical from life as I'd known it thus far. While most students had full-time jobs lined up after graduation, my plan had always been to travel first through Britain and Europe. I tried to keep telling myself I was running toward, not away from, myself — a concept Morgan had instilled in me. I actually prayed before leaving that I would be rid of my moodiness and bodily abuse, and embrace the peace of mind and body Dianna had talked about. I prepared a makeshift will, leaving much of my writing journals to Pam. The night before I left, my well-travelled friend Susan came over, and gave me a pep talk and the names of numerous friends in various countries to contact if I ever needed a place to stay. She gave me a strong hug, and told me I was about to have the time of my life. The following morning, when my friend Sharon arrived with a journal and travel alarm clock, we sat on my parents' porch and shared a box of Kleenex. Tears were also shed with my parents at the airport, but once the plane left the ground, I was flying.

By and large, the momentum of self-esteem I had managed to muster in the sanctity of my own apartment flourished overseas. It was an infinite growing experience, brimming with discovery, creativity, and self-expression; a time when I had no choice but to try and make peace with myself. The eyes tell the story of that success — they were alive with a sparkle previously unknown. The high seas, the mountains, the culture, the freedom; all proved to be the tonic I'd forever sought. I experienced the world in a way beyond even my wildest dreams. Cycling alongside sheep against the remote beauty on the Isle of Skye. Watching the White Cliffs of Dover disappear, as the fine Belgian shore beckoned on the horizon. Imagining myself the young, terrified Anne Frank, closeted away, furiously journalizing her world before meeting her fate in a tiny Amsterdam house. Dwarfed by centuries-old *tannenbaums* in the Black Forest. Wending my way through the time-warped bleak and barren streets of East Berlin. Cleansing old wounds in the idyllic beauty of Interlaaken and Mutters. Waking to bustling rue Mouffetard outside my Paris hostel room. Standing dumbfounded beneath the Leaning Tower of Pisa. Gazing out across the vast Atlantic, from the Portuguese tip of Sagres, as had new world dreamers da Gama and Henry the Navigator before me. Exploring Cretan ruins under the watchful eye of gentle Greek goddesses. Seduced by Istanbul's mournful calls to mosque. Kicking back for a month of hippiedom on the beaches of Taba, the infamous "no-man's land" between Israel and Egypt.

But for a handful of relapses, bulimia reared not its ugly head. Not to be fooled, my drinking escalated, as I savoured the thrill of going deeper into myself than I had ever allowed. My well-trodden feet crossed paths with those from all corners of the world: from Sweden to Australia, from Chile to Japan, we were strangers bound by a common thirst for travel. Whether sharing cramped and freezing quarters in dead-of-winter Belgrade, working the fields on a kibbutz in the Golan Heights, huddled around a campfire in the Negev desert, drinking red wine well past sunset in France, or tasting sea spray on the deck of a ferryboat, they knew nothing of me, nor I of them. Yet still we bonded, in that kindred sort of way, weaving ourselves into the tapestry of each other's lives. They validated my existence, accepting my presence, not questioning my past or my future. There was no need to hide behind a mask. I cautiously began to see myself without it.

In spite of the rivers of local wine and beer I consumed as I made my way through country after country, pencils, pens, and notebooks were my constant companions. I took pleasure in scribing voluminous letters to friends, sharing the wonders of my newly discovered world. Strangely enough, I also wrote in veritable opus-style to my parents, the distance between us my ally. To the friends and family I'd gradually and painstakingly cocooned away from during my teens and early twenties, it was a world seen through the eyes of a stranger that burst out of the envelope. Caught in the rolls of photos I sent home for developing, my eyes were brimming with the blessings of the world. I'd never felt so good about myself, content with my life. I was free. Never was that feeling so powerful than when I made my way up to the top of Switzerland's Mount Pilatus, where I lay on the snow-capped, sun-drenched summit, as pillows of serenity clouds drifted almost within reach.

But in sharp contrast to the self-nurturing of my European journey, returning to Canada in August 1987 constituted a huge setback; old wounds salted with a vengeance I'd forfeited a year earlier greeted me. As if trapped in an ongoing nightmare, I roamed the streets of Hamilton, a displaced veteran of wonderful travels, ravaged by the feeling I did not belong. Living back with my parents, I felt stripped of the individuality I had worked so hard to let flourish, suffocated in a repressive straitjacket of conformity and emptiness. Contrary to the detailed letters I had written them from overseas, I had no desire to walk them through my trip, country by country, in such close proximity, beneath the same roof. The door I had opened for them to walk through via correspondence was virtually slammed shut when I returned. They were naturally confused to say the least, for I seemed to be living two lives that were in constant friction with each other.

In January 1988, we all had a reprieve from the nothingness of my being when I was offered the opportunity to house-sit for my friend Trisha's parents. I jumped at the chance. It was precisely the refuge I needed. Nevertheless, I was afraid that so much time alone would prove unwise. For the most part, my social contact after I moved some clothes, books, and journals into their home was limited to the three part-time jobs I juggled to rebuild my bank account before heading off to graduate school at Montreal's McGill University in the fall. As I'd feared, my time was otherwise spent succumbing to drinking and eating patterns more destructive than ever within the confines of a house all to myself.

In returning to Hamilton, I was living a nightmare; unwittingly finding myself back on the passive suicidal train barrelling into the longest and darkest of days. By early March, I was at the end of my tether, having virtually cleaned out fridge, freezer, and cupboards of all food and liquor. I vomitted almost every morsel of food I ate. I soothed my raw and ragged throat with tumblers full of rye whiskey on ice. Blood-shot and puffy eyes stared back from every mirror I passed by and dared to look at. *"Nancy with the laughing eyes,"* as my Grandma Reid often referred to me when I was a child, had been left overseas.

Twenty-two: Too little too late

"... but rest and peace were still denied him, so he finally put an end to his misery by drowning himself."

[MARK TWAIN — *A Tramp Abroad*]

BY THE TIME I returned home from Europe, five years had passed since Mom had been stabilized on lithium. In the space of a few harrowing months back at home, I had regressed whereby I was no better a daughter than I had been prior to, or at the beginning of, her emergence into relative wellness in November 1982. I was thrust back to my shadowy elusive self; barely a daughter at all. I was trapped between wanting to be supportive to Mom, and suffocating under the weight of the pressure to do so. At times, I felt barely human, for the way I ravaged my body was as a wild animal that had never been adequately nourished. For insomuch as she died when I was born, and for as long as I had lived in the shadow of her death, I was none the wiser about how to live. Each day back on Canadian soil had me grasping at the threads that made up the tattered fabric of my life; sadly, the barest patches of all were the ones my mother had been unable to tightly weave for — for either of us — all those years ago. And how sad that even though I had the knowledge that she was now more living than dying, I could not rid myself of the premature death she had suffered. I was born of a fabric that struggled to live while she was dying and was bent on sowing the seeds of my own death while she was living. There was nothing worth harvesting. Knowledge means nothing, when so little comes so late.

Perhaps the saving grace for Mom after she came out of the hospital and the years that followed, with a husband in reactive depression, a son out of town, and a daughter out of touch, was the support she received beyond our family. Through Dr. Reimer, the psychiatrist at St. Joseph's, she became involved with a social worker by the name of Margaret Keller. In addition to regular meetings with her, Mom also became part of Margaret's small support group for women on lithium. With a core of about six members, they would meet for two hours every Thursday afternoon down at St. Joseph's Hospital to discuss what was going on in their lives. After two decades of suffering in isolation, surrounded by people who did not understand what she was going through, Mom finally had the opportunity to share her experiences with other women and hear stories similar to hers.

Still, she was a minority in the group. Most women were diagnosed as having bipolar disorder, and recounted tales of manic episodes beyond the scope of anything Mom could identify with. Inevitably, the group dynamics were not always conducive to each person having time to speak as much as she needed each week. As Mom is shy by nature, the more extroverted ones tended to dominate discussions. Yet if she was tentative about being part of such a group, she never let on and attended the weekly sessions religiously. The therapeutic value of feeling less alone, guilty, and ashamed of the past outweighed any reservations she may have had. As the various members of the group changed, she remained a constant, from 1982 until Margaret Keller's retirement some ten years later.

Although I would often acknowledge Mom's weekly meetings, I was equally careful to respect her privacy. I was sure that within the safety of the group structure, she could talk about things she never could or would with our family or close friends. Admittedly, my interest in Mom's group also extended to the other members, and how their lives, not unlike Mom's, had been ravaged by cruel and relentless moodswings. Did they have children? Did they ever discuss the effect of their illness upon them? Would there ever be a chance for me to meet Margaret Keller and the other women in the group? After years of feeling our family was an island in the storms of depression, I harboured a thirst to speak with others similarly affected. Although I had heard about and met other patients in the hospital psychiatric wards over the years, this was a different need — perhaps because I was older and more cognizant of the damage depression had bestowed upon our family.

On one occasion in the mid 1980s, I did meet two of the women when they drove Mom home from their weekly meeting. As I was being introduced to Rose and Bernice, it was all I could do to choke back the tears and swallow my heart from where it threatened to leap out of my mouth. Bernice was a divorced mother of an 11-year-old girl named Molly. Without even knowing either of them, my heart ached for her daughter and the loneliness of living in the uncertainty of her mother's manic depression without another parent or sibling to cushion the blow. At least Dad had stayed, and I'd had Barry. I wanted to offer to this little girl what Barry and I never had: someone to talk to; to let her know she wasn't alone. Periodically, I'd muse aloud to Mom about being a big sister of sorts to Molly. But neither Mom nor I took the initiative to pursue the idea with Bernice, thereby perpetuating the myth that offspring and partners are secondary sufferers who will somehow find their own way.

It was not until late 1987 that I finally met Margaret Keller and Dr. Reimer, the two people who had been instrumental in Mom's recovery, when Mom and I attended a forum on manic depression. Although Mom never suffered mania, it was an opportunity I dared not miss, if I was ever to gain access to the secret world Mom had so long inhabited.

The facilitator was psychiatrist Dr. Nate Kerwin, a tall, lean man with a very unassuming demeanour and a hint of a British accent. One of the key issues raised by Dr. Kerwin was the lack of therapy, education, and support for the families of persons with mood disorders. He acknowledged that treatment is individual-specific, and thereby negates the affectation of significant others. He spoke of the long-term effect on attachment between mother and child and the impact on child development, particularly if the depression begins with postpartum episodes. When the mother is ill and especially if hospitalized, the newborn is deprived of requisite nurturing. As the children grow up, they will need to cope with the parents' illness in a way that may cause them to become parents in their own family, taking care of household chores, looking after the sick parent, and being good kids. Although living with a depressed parent can help children to mature quickly, it is often at the expense of their own well-being, as the spirit of childhood slips through their fingers.

I couldn't believe my ears. He was speaking directly to me. For more than 20 years I had been waiting to hear something like this: a corroboration of our family's story; that all those years we had not been making mountains out of mere molehills, as Mom's doctors had too often led us to believe.

In order to comprehend the magnitude of depression and mania, Dr. Kerwin stressed that the illness must be understood in terms of environment and the people therein. It is imperative, he noted, that family members understand that the illness is the fault of nobody. He advocated a more collaborative approach between doctors and family members, with the hope that those closest would be more attuned to changes in the person at the onset of each cycle of the illness. In so doing, there would be a better chance of getting ahead of the disorder, so that it could be treated on an outpatient basis as opposed to hospitalization, which, as Dr. Kerwin pointed out, is extremely disruptive to the family structure, and is often met with significant client resistance.

From time to time, I sneaked a peek around the room. Everyone appeared so uninterested. I felt I could have exploded. So much to say, so many questions. Where to start? I ached to stand up and scream "YES!" and to share with the others and Dr. Kerwin our family's experience. But the longer I squirmed in my hard wooden seat, the more I became increasingly aware of how structured and clinical the setting was — not remotely conducive to spilling out my thoughts and feelings after all. Suddenly, I was like an uninvited guest. Most people present were in couples, and one boy of about 12 sat glumly between two adults. It was a safe guess that we were the token mother-daughter team. I refrained from speaking, suppressing everything deeper inside.

After Dr. Kerwin's presentation, at the very least, I was hoping to meet Margaret Keller and Dr. Reimer. As it was, they were both speaking together when Mom and I walked over to them. When she introduced me, I was disappointed that it didn't seem terribly important that I was there with Mom, even though none of the other women from her support group was present. I was sure that Margaret Keller would at least thank me for the Christmas cards I had sent her, acknowledging her role and that of the group in Mom's continued wellness. But neither she nor Dr. Reimer paid me much heed beyond a brief "hello" as I stood dumbly beside Mom. Who did I think I was anyway, expecting more than I was getting? I chided myself for being so needy, for admittedly, I'd been hoping to have someone ask how I was doing and how I had managed over the years of Mom's illness. Maybe I'd even meet someone whose mother had also had hundreds of shock treatments. Ironically, both Margaret and Dr. Reimer were reinforcing everything that Dr. Kerwin had just described as lacking: communication with and support for family members.

Where the forum had started out inflating my hopes of gaining insight into our family dynamics, it left me hanging in mid-air. At least I had gained somewhat of a confirmation that as a family, we had been dealt a lousy hand, and began to understand why we were having such an uphill struggle with the success of lithium. For the previous five years we had been blindly forging ahead, grateful with each day, week, month, and year that Mom was well. To some degree, the forum was a misplaced piece of the puzzle confirming in my mind that it had always been too little too late.

That night I remembered something I had not thought of in years: acting "retarded." There was a period when I was about 10 years old, when I would be overcome with an urge to be close to my Mom. Oddly enough, this would happen when we were downtown shopping together. I have a clear memory of us walking down King William Street, not a busy stretch, but certainly not empty of people or shops. It was the route I preferred, emerging out the back door of the "lower class" Kresges to make our way over to the more prestigious Eatons. Without any warning, I would grab Mom's arm and pretend to be "retarded." I would cling ever so tightly, leaning into her side as I walked with a pronounced limp. I'd hang my tongue out of my open mouth, and droop my lids lazily over my eye lids. I knew that if I looked "retarded," I could get away with holding on to her and people wouldn't think it foolish at my age. It didn't matter to me that people often look with rude curiosity at such deviations from the norm. The need to be close to my Mom, albeit in such an awkward and obtuse way, was what mattered. It worked. Much as she tried to squirm away, laughing nervously and telling me to stop, the sad reality is that she would allow me to act like that, if only for a block or two. Did she too miss the tactile comfort that should be inherent in a mother-daughter relationship?

When I looked around the room that night, I wondered if any other kids had ever clung to a parent like that. Would anybody understand? Did Mom remember that?

Of course I never asked her. Unfortunately, neither did I make the opportunity to talk about the evening much with Mom, let alone Dad or Barry. Nevertheless, hearing what I did that night about mental illness put so much in perspective, particularly the reason for our apparent failure to suddenly become a perfect, close-knit family once Mom was better. Our reality proved far from that fairytale optimism. Our family network had long ago eroded, beneath a thin coat of veneer. Had I not been so hell-bent on my own self-destruction over the years, perhaps the erosion may not have been quite so devastating. Finding our way back to one another was virtually like starting a family from scratch. For what was there to go back to? And even if there was a place from which we could reasonably begin again, I for one was too busy dying.

against the odds

two turtle doves
same branch
different limb
looking out toward tomorrow
as the colour of the day
breathes hope of a common wish
for the health
of the mind and body . . .

Part III: Into the fire

Twenty-three: Seoul to soul

We share the same spit-covered, garbage-littered streets; we breathe the same exhaust-gutted air spewed from the cars of johns, who cruise the battered and stoned ladies of the night by day. We are hostage to the yellow-eyed pimps who prowl; but we are safe in our own little world . . .

BY THE GRACE of a far eastern wind, I had somewhat of a reprieve from my invasive terror of being when I met a woman by the name of Yunee on March 12, 1988. The day was bitter cold and icy. The Friday night before, I had arrived in Toronto to spend the weekend with our mutual friend Pam. When I was introduced to Yunee the following afternoon, I was suffering the ill-effects of one too many glasses of red wine and too many tears cried the night previous; my head was virtually held atop my shoulders with a swaddling of scarves. She still teases me about being garbed in a second-hand *Colombo*-like trench coat fastened together by a few safety pins and sporting shortish hair with a wild mess of gel; essentially, the physical attire was merely a reflection of the owner's emotional instability.

Nevertheless, between glasses of Soave white wine and bottles of Fosters lager, she defied my shy, evasive looks, and captivated me with her easy-going playfulness and eyes that danced in time with the flames in the fireplace behind her. As fate would govern, we never looked back after that night. A native of Seoul, South Korea, Yunee came into my life at a time when I was virtually scraping the bottom of the emotional, mental, and physical bucket; I felt ruined, held together by the very pins that secured my coat. Though my own prognosis for recovery had been slim to nil, there was a flicker of renewed hope for the safety-pinned soul who was clinging to the edge of something called life.

As our relationship flourished, I foolishly assumed my reckless eating and drinking patterns would disappear. I presented Yunee with a chestnut-brown leather mask that I'd purchased from a street vendor in Lisbon; a gesture symbolic of my refusal to hide behind false faces any longer. Were it only so easy, we would have been spared many hurtful days and nights. But my demons shadowed me during my furtive commutes to Yunee's west-end Toronto apartment. I agonized over how I was betraying her, for she knew not of the self-destructive veins tunnelling beneath my skin. I shielded her from myself as I did everyone, fearing she would take the high road and leave me in a heap along the dusty shoulder. To the contrary, when I finally revealed my ongoing struggle with food, a portion of the wall between us crumbled. Only then could we begin to move forward through the rubble.

Nevertheless, I could not bring myself to reveal the extent to which eating ruled my life. How could I explain the terror that consumed me each time Yunee left for work? I was afraid to be alone in her apartment on the weekends that I stayed over, for I knew the minute she was out the door, I would revert to my ritualistic intake of food. I cringe to think of what she must have noticed at the time, but did not know how to discuss with me, for even her career as a registered nurse had not prepared her for dealing with an eating disorder. For the most part, we carried on, enraptured as we were with the newness of our relationship and the complexities of discovering each other's world.

The more I revealed myself to Yunee, however, the more I concealed from friends and family the life I was building beyond the reaches of Hamilton. Moving in with Yunee July 31, 1988, alleviated the burden of lies for my weekly forays into Toronto, but raised more questions about my mysterious "room-mate." Nevertheless, I explained our living arrangement as one of convenience. When my parents dropped me off at the Hamilton bus terminal with my few belongings, I think there was relief mixed with apprehension all around. Since returning from Europe the previous summer, my parents had borne the brunt of my aloofness and moodiness. My life was lived in a tangled web of white lies that I consistently spun in order to protect them, especially Mom, from the true nature of their daughter. In the back of my mind, I still haboured a fear of Mom relapsing. I was certain that my relationship with Yunee would trigger her depression, which continued to be in remission. Though I had always been torn by the need to be free of my parents' home in the name of self-preservation, I had been equally compelled to stay to look after Mom, acting as a buffer between my parents. But since my return from overseas, I had rarely been there physically for her, and certainly not emotionally. Now, my parents would have to do without me. I don't know if any of us knew how long it would take me to ever return.

Living in Toronto, I began to taste the freedom and selfhood that I'd savoured through Europe not so very long ago. I loved the walks with Yunee down to the lakefront we could see from our balcony, my weekend pilgrimages along Roncesvalles Avenue and Bloor Street when Yunee was at work, and becoming part of Toronto and of our Parkdale neighbourhood in a way that grounded me in a new reality. Despite its reputation as one of the city's less desirable environs, I felt strangely at home on this turf of the dispossessed.

Within a month, I landed a bilingual administrative position for a national non-profit association within walking distance from our apartment. Things seemed to be falling into place, when I began to feel myself slipping back into the arms of an all-familiar weighted blur. Working 12 hours a day to tackle the legacy of previous employees, I seemed to be no further ahead in my workload. By mid-October, crying spells began to occur at work for no apparent reason. I was granted a couple of days off to collect myself. Though the phase was short-lived, it was a warning sign that all was not well. Nevertheless, I was soon swimming up the stream of productive workaholism, which would see me rewarded me with a promotion to membership services coordinator before year-end.

In November 1988, Mom and I celebrated her sixth year of wellness. I quietly commemorated the six years since the onset of my eating disorder. I congratulated myself that the purging had been in remission for eight days, and dared to wonder if I was finally out of the woods. But I was never far from an undergrowth of gloom, which tripped me up time and again. The next wave of crippling darkness washed over me seemingly unannounced in March 1989. I was attending a strategic planning session with staff and members of the board, when I tuned into a sinking, foreboding sensation, overwhelmed by the magnitude of goals and objectives we were discussing. I could feel my self-esteem and confidence draining away from me. I felt lost in the maze of expectations and idealisms that I perceived as being heaped on to me and me alone. The next day, I called in sick, thinking I just needed a couple of extra days to re-group and re-energize myself for the work ahead.

That pattern repeated itself; my dependability on the job was at stake, as time-sensitive projects were jeopardized and colleagues had to take over some of my work. At the onset of such an episode, my thought processes slowed and my clarity of issues was veiled. On one occasion, while orientating a colleague about a component of my job I was handing over to him, I was unable to convey the necessary and routine information. Tears rather than words came forth. Excusing myself, I fled to the washroom. It was starting all over.

Sleeping more. Don't want to get up. Drinking more. Eating more. Unable to concentrate. Overwhelmed by the routine of the day. At that point, I decided to speak with Dr. Catherine Wong, the family physician I'd hooked up with when I first moved to Toronto. Though the signs and symptoms were present, I never considered myself to be depressed in the medical sense of the term. That was reserved for Mom, a condition that I could not rightfully assume for myself. Much to my dismay, Dr. Wong prescribed antidepressants. The hell with that, I thought to myself, as I sat teary-eyed before her. Five bucks and a doctor's note later, I pleaded my case to my sympathetic boss, Susan, for a few days off sick. Once again, I was permitted time away without ever being able to pinpoint what was wrong. When I walked the streets of Parkdale, I felt as if I belonged. Though I was not one of the throngs of de-institutionalized souls who gravitate to that part of Toronto, I was living among them by choice — the only difference being I didn't have to scrimp for a morning muffin; I still had a job.

Somehow, I was always given chances to go back to work, wholly due to my sympathetic managers Mark and Susan, who were able to separate my feast of productivity during the "good times" from the relative famine during the downswings. For that I was grateful, for I loved the writing and editing components my job had expanded to include. But each time I returned, I sensed people were walking on eggshells, uncertain of the waters around me. Over the years my other colleagues Manon, Catherine, Silvia, Gerry, and Claudia were stead-fast beacons through my many storms, for as a small staff, we became very much a family-like entity, and fostered friendships that have endured ever since. Though time and again calm skies eventually prevailed, fear and uncertainty hovered, with me never knowing when and why the slumps kept recurring.

Stress is a common precipitating factor in depression. The more adept one is at handling stress, the less chance for depression to set in. Yet when depressed, there is less chance that stress can be handled. In retrospect, I had a history of identifiable trigger points that preceded my depressions as far back as high school. In the late 1970s and early '80s, Mom's illness and my parents incessant arguing clashed with my issues of low self-esteem, sexuality, alcohol, and food. By the late 1980s and early 1990s, relationship turbulence caused me considerable grief. The primary agitator with Yunee was my habit of 10- to 12-hour workdays — inconceivable to a registered nurse who is not required to stay on the floor when her eight-hour shift is over. Though my bulimia had been pretty much in remission since November 1988, my excessive drinking binges also ignited significant friction between Yunee and me.

Though the reality of intimate relationships is that discord will inevitably arise, when Yunee and I were at odds with each other, it was as if my whole world collapsed. Both Yunee and I were raised in homes where parental feuding was commonplace; neither of us learned "healthy arguing." In my mind, disputes were synonymous with anger and had no place in my life without mortally wounding another. Our quibbles were often exacerbated because we were quite insular, depending on each other for all physical and emotional needs, not revealing the nature of our relationship to most others around us. The strain of leading a double life, closeted away from family, co-workers, and many friends, was taking its toll on both of us. Nevertheless, we persevered, and in January 1990, moved from our Parkdale apartment overlooking the lake to our first home backing onto a ravine in the wilds of southwest Etobicoke.

[MARCH 1990 — JOURNAL ENTRY] *Dragging self up from the deep recesses of the bed, dreading the thought of the day. Unable to cope at work; brain not functioning. Concentration zip; creative juices dried up; thoughts lost to vacant haze of memory. Feel so low ...*

In March 1990, the stress of homeownership was complicated by a relationship crisis that sent me plummeting to new lows. My drinking escalated and many times I was either too hung-over to make it to work, or too fuzzy to concentrate while I was there. For the better part of a month, I was off sick, during which time, Dr. Wong once again advised antidepressants. I was uncomfortable with the relative ease with which she seemed willing to do so. How could she be so sure such an extreme measure was necessary? On the previous occasions in the past year and a half when I had felt down, I had discussed with her my reluctance to take medication. With an almost what-the-hell attitude, I went through the motions of filling the prescription for Imipramine. The mere presence of that little unopened bottle in my medicine chest conjured up a flood of ambivalence until it took its rightful place in the trash several years later. I resolved to change my doctor.

Throughout my employment with the non-profit association, the cycles of depression were interspersed with windows of opportunity when my writing and editing skills were worthy of merit and even pride. For the most part, I enjoyed my job, and the relationships formed with colleagues and members alike. When I departed in August 1992 in quest of a new career challenge, I did not let myself be daunted by the risk presented by being unemployed. By the end of September, I'd landed a contract position with Metro Toronto Community Services as a communications coordinator for a provincial job-training program. The job description was intimidating to say the least. My contact for the position was Susan, my former manager, whom I was surprised would consider me a worthy candidate, given her knowledge of my attendance history. Nevertheless, I was interviewed and hired within a matter of days.

My good fortune with the job coincided with running my first marathon, a feat to which I had long aspired and had committed myself to accomplish the year I turned 30. Completing the 26.2-mile course in just under four hours inspired in me a confidence for the challenge of the career path ahead. Mentally and physically, I was in better shape than I had ever been.

[OCTOBER 1992 — JOURNAL ENTRY] *Feeling really down. Overwhelmed. Emotionally out of control. Want to scream or throw something. Bile builds, head throbs — if I drink will it go away? Feel small. Dragging myself from bed to get last bus. How will I make it through the day? Want to close off the world except for Yunee and my dog C.C. They are my salvation. Scared, choked by visions of inadequacy, losing it all. Want to sob. Crippled. Unable to do anything. No food. Not even coffee. Somehow carrying on . . .*

By early November 1992, I was swept back into the cave of unremitting darkness. Saddled with work responsibilities that were rife with political nuances, my mind and body told me I was in over my head. With no visible light at the end of the tunnel, I succumbed to the familiar pattern of calling in sick, unable to fathom tackling the reams of paperwork, committee reports, and correspondence that awaited me. The lower I sank, the clearer it became I would have to leave, for I had lost all confidence in my ability to carry on. When I discussed the decision with my managers Susan and Deborah, it was acknowledged that I was being stretched beyond the limits of what I'd been hired to do. I was given a few days off to refresh myself and asked to reconsider leaving, with assurances that my job would be streamlined in a more manageable fashion. Though part of me was relieved to know my downward turn was beyond my reasonable control, I was alarmed that I had succumbed so quickly in a new job. Yet again, I had been reigned in from the brink of total collapse.

Twenty-four: Running on empty

[DECEMBER 24, 1993 — JOURNAL ENTRY] *When will I stop running? And from what? The ultimate running away. I want to be sick. What is this bug in my brain that causes so much pain. I am dead in the head. I am tormenting us both to death . . .*

THROUGH 1993, the periods of wellness were staggered by recurring bouts of profound melancholia during January, March, July, August, November, and December. My alcohol consumption was also increasing with undesirable consequences on my relationship, particularly when I went out with colleagues after work and made it home just before Yunee at 11:00 p.m. Slightly drunk on the day's diet of copious cups of coffee, a muffin, and several quickly imbibed beers, I was famished and far from capable of carrying on meaningful conversation, though we would have not seen each other all day. Caught up once again in 10- or 12-hour workdays, my sense of priority and selfhood was slipping from my grasp. I was dancing with the devils of doom and gloom yet again.

In July, I became involved with the "Guided Self-Change Program" at the Addiction Research Foundation (ARF), for people concerned about their alcohol use. Based on the concept of guided self-change, the objective is to help clients identify problem drinking situations and establish goals around drinking behaviour, whether that be defined as total abstinence or moderation. My aim was to have more control over the occasions when I succumbed to excessive drinking. Long-term abstinence did not seem realistic to me; in fact, the thought of never drinking again was incomprehensible. I had never gone for much more than a week without a drink in the past 15 years. My goal was to set guidelines for myself within which to drink safely. For the first couple of months in the program, I struggled to curtail the problem situations. Focusing on them did not, however, preclude their happening, but at least I had the support of a wonderful counsellor in her early 60s by the name of Joan Bradley, with whom to discuss them and better understand them. Many tears were cried as I talked about my job and relationship anxieties, in addition to the seemingly constant battle with the bottle. On more than one occasion, the issue of depression was raised. Though I sure felt down in the dumps, I was not comfortable with referring to myself as depressive.

In December 1993, I experienced what I refer to as a "bottoming out." Over dinner with a colleague three days before Christmas, a bottle of wine, and hours later, I stumbled through the door drunk as a skunk and faced the music with Yunee, who, understandably, was thinking the worst of all possible angles, about where the hell I had been. That evening caused near irrevocable damage to the-then fragile equilibrium between my partner and me, as my all-consuming job and colleague outings left me with only the residue of emotional energy for our relationship. And it would get worse before it got better, as I slipped into a tailspin from December through into March 1994. My life was an out-of-control roller coaster. After countless derailments over the years, it was as if I was experiencing the impact of all of the previous crashes.

Resolving to pick up the pieces yet again, I began the New Year in search of a therapist with whom I could somehow sort out the tattered pieces of my life. Though I was still working with Joan at ARF to address alcohol issues, we agreed I needed to go beyond that scope to address the deep-rooted crazy-making nature of my life. After investigating several newspaper listings, making quick phone calls from behind the closed door of my office, I spoke with Claire Richardson, a private counsellor with expertise, among other areas, in addiction, recovery, and relationship issues. Something in her voice immediately set her apart from the other women with whom I'd spoken. Though initially taken aback by her frank personal details ("I'm a 41-year-old 'dyke,' and have been clean and sober for nine years"), I found myself contriving an excuse to leave work early and head out to her east-end apartment-cum-office.

Once her heavenly brewed java cut through my anxiety as I perched ready to take flight from her couch, we connected on some level, and not only because we were both native Hamiltonians. Her "been there, done that" attitude assured me I could risk brutal honesty about the gory details of my life without fear of judgement. For an hour or so a week, I felt saner and somewhat grounded. Fifty dollars a session was a comparably small price to pay for intermittent doses of sanity. But beyond the security of our sessions, I was barely treading water in the murky waters of despondency. In constant conflict with Yunee, I spent an inordinate amount of time thinking I should just blow my head off; yet thankful we didn't own a gun.

It's safe to say that my counsellors Joan and Claire were polar opposites. This was never more apparent than the time the three of us met at Joan's office, so that each could get a sense of how the other was dealing with my issues around addiction. Joan's approach to addiction and what she perceived as my depression was more academic and clinical, in a sense. But her compassionate nature and soft-spoken ways nurtured me in an almost motherly manner. By contrast, Claire's own life experiences provided a framework for her counselling in the realm of addiction, recovery, and relationship issues. It was a strange experience for me, at times feeling caught in the middle between two therapists who were both trying to treat the same problem: me. My job was to extract the best of both models and not lose my head in the process.

As January dragged into February, professionally, I was paralyzed by an ever-present fear of incompetence. I was afraid colleagues would see through me, that I was a fraud and not at all suited to a work culture that indirectly condoned 14- to 16-hour days and demanded increasing political savvy and bureaucratic thick skin. My insecurity evolved into a jagged rock that gouged holes in my stomach, creating a pit I was helpless to fill. Before long, I was barely able to crawl out of bed before 7:00 a.m. to make the painful 15-minute GO-train trek downtown.

Withering under the scrutiny of all the corporate types scanning their perfectly folded newspapers, I averted the world behind my haven of dark sunglasses on even the greyest of mornings. Once at the office, I kept my door closed and was uncomfortably aware that my colleagues were warily keeping their distance when I emerged, unsure whether to speak or make eye contact. I hated myself for what was happening. I was shrouded in a fog so thick it distorted my thought processes and left my concentration capacity in shreds. Though the transformation may have been sudden to those around me, I experienced it as a progressive journey to deep dark depths. I struggled to hang on, but my grip was ever weakening. A mere five days during the month of March 1994 did I make it to work, opting most days to bury my head into the pillow, wishing I had a hatchet with which to cut it off. I was a hollow mass drifting from day to day.

Sucked into the depths, even my usual salvation of running several miles caused my chest to tighten in a way that I feared the mitral-valve prolapse I'd been diagnosed with some 10 years earlier was getting the better of me. When I'd become winded doing slight jogs up two or three flights of stairs, I knew I was in real trouble, like a rusted generator, void of the weakest of power surges. I tortured myself with the chicken-and-egg riddle: was I feeling so lousy because of my job and relationship, or were those problems symptomatic of an ongoing gloominess some called depression? Life was eating me up and I had all but swallowed myself whole.

Twenty-five: Shrink-wrapped puddles

"I came to the puddle. I could not cross it. Identity failed me. Then very gingerly, I pushed my foot across. I laid my back against a brick wall. I returned very painfully, drawing myself back into my body over the grey cadaverous space in the puddle. This is the life then to which I am committed."

[VIRGINIA WOOLF — *The Waves*]

DURING THE eight months I had been meeting with Joan, on more than one occasion, she questioned whether I was not clinically depressed. As I sat in her office, tears streaming down my face, she gently tried to encourage me to give medication a chance and suggested I speak with Dr. Seymour Kane, the resident ARF psychiatrist. If her guess was correct, and I was "depressed," there were medications that could help me. Each time she broached the subject, a warning bell clanged in my head: no psychiatrists and certainly no medication. Though Joan understood my resistance was based on my family's experiences over the years, she tried to encourage me to reconsider, summoning the analogy that, if I were diabetic, I'd have to take insulin, wouldn't I? Knowing how Mom needs to be on lithium for the rest of her life, the thought of falling prey to a similar fate was out of the question. Nevertheless, by early March 1994, as the weight of the demon named darkness in my head tipped the scales unmercifully in favour of succumbing to nothingness, I surrendered, agreeing to meet with Dr. Kane, at least for an assessment.

[TUESDAY, MARCH 8, 1994 — JOURNAL ENTRY] *International Women's Day. 8:35 a.m. train in for 9:30 a.m. meeting with Dr. Kane, the "label maker." How many people on this train are happy about where they are going? I'm living in a way I don't want to live. Same script. Head heavy and don't want to deal with life. Shut self off. Want to run because I'm not functioning. Walking from Union Station up to ARF. The waiting room. Waiting for a shrink. Quiet of ARF so fucking sterile. Visions of St. Joe's; Henderson. Visiting Mom. Calculated laughter echoes from somewhere. Watching sparrows fly in and around a church steeple visible outside. Joan briefing Dr. Kane. "I'll go get the chart." I hear her say, adding, "Doesn't tell you much." Footsteps. Back again. Door closes. Muffled drone of voices. The hamster on the rotator. More like a rat today. What the hell am I doing here . . .*

I admit to harbouring less than favourable notions about psychiatrists, and Dr. Kane did nothing to dispel my preconceived ideas. His dishevelled appearance reflected the disarray in his cubby hole of an office: file folders strewn upon every available surface; empty Styrofoam coffee cups, brown plastic stir-sticks, and discarded sugar packets littered the desk and floor. Arms folded, he hunched over the desk, and questioned me with an unsettling quirkiness. Sitting across from him, my leather coat zipped to the neck, I was ready to take flight at any moment, skeptical that the clutter of his office could breed any logic to the muddle of my mind. Nothing about him conveyed professionalism or instilled any confidence that this guy knew what he was doing. To make matters worse, his mannerisms, voice, and features mimicked those of a guy from Hamilton who had stalked me a few years previous. Spooked and distracted, I did my best to respond to his questions dutifully, describing the world in which I lived.

Feeling depressed on and off for past eight months. Sinking deeper and deeper. Sleeping too much. Stomach juices pumping round the clock. Spewing bile in the morning. Erratic eating. Listless. Crying. Unable to concentrate. Job in jeopardy. Reclusive. Cholesterol elevated to 8.6. Heart aches. Winded when walking. Running an ordeal.

Genetics. Mom depressed 20 years. Lithium levelled for 12. Dad depressed too. Medication. Alcohol abuse and me a recurring theme. Bulimic six years. In remission for five years with periodic relapses.

Within an hour, the depression diagnosis suspected months earlier by Joan was confirmed by Dr. Kane. Citing two primary causes of clinical depression, biological and circumstantial, in my case, he suspected it could be a combination of both. Family history and the recurring nature of my cycles of depression pointed to a significant genetic component. Crises in my life suggested situational triggers characterized by my physical symptoms and current mental state. He recommended medication immediately. I paled. Antidepressants, he said. Stunned. He's serious. Cannot believe I actually need medication. Tricyclics. Selective serotonin reuptake inhibitors (SSRIs). Lots of options, he reassured me. Head spinning. Visions of Mom. pillspillspillspillspills.

Staring beyond him to the cream-coloured wall, made dizzy by the pattern of dried Scotch Tape marks streaked upon them. I listened as he proclaimed I was a prime candidate for Prozac. I flinched. Dad's Prozac past had turned ugly. Night sweats, nightmares, severe mood swings. But Dr. Kane didn't miss a beat. Depression, alcoholism, and bulimia — all related to same neurotransmitter: serotonin, he specified. That struck a nerve. My friend Pam had once recommended a book written about the serotonin connection. He continued. Prozac regulates serotonin levels in brain. Combats all three. "Dual diagnosis," he called it; something about me having both a mood disorder and substance-abuse problems. Wouldn't that be great? Nab all the demons in one fell swoop. My thoughts or his voice: mine drip with dread; his oozes sterile enthusiasm.

But I was not to be swayed. I did not want to take medication. I'd witnessed Mom and then Dad go through dozens of prescriptions that led nowhere. I also knew of neighbours and a couple of friends who were caught in the revolving door of depression, drugs, and side effects. Picking up on where I was headed, Dr. Kane admitted antide-pressants have received their share of bad press. He tried to assure me that Prozac and other SSRIs were different; and though they could be overused, they could also be lifesavers, once the right one was identi-fied as being compatible.

Finding the "right one" opened the door to my next fear: side effects. I did not want anything that would change my personality, cause weight gain, cold sweats, dizziness, dry mouth, or any number of things I knew were common unpleasantries of antidepressants. The longer the trial-and-error phase, the greater the chance of adverse effects, he seemed to be saying. In my mind, antidepressants were syn-onymous with the loss of my creative self, being split off from my essence. Nevertheless, Dr. Kane assured me that side effects would be monitored and that I had nothing to fear. Furthermore, the likelihood of success was high because the molecular abnormalities were genetic. Parrotting Joan's diabetes analogy, he impressed that chemicals in anti-depressants modulate mood just as insulin regulates diabetes. Perhaps only a six-month trial period would be necessary to help me better deal with situations, he assured. Whereas now I could not work, soon I would be able to resume a level of productivity, he predicted.

That Dr. Kane was clearly having no qualms about prescribing antidepressants so readily was somewhat unsettling. A faint voice of virtue decried the ethics of antidepressants being so easily prescribed, giving substance to the parallel of Prozac as the Valium of the '90s. While I never associated antidepressants with weakness and failure for my parents and friends, they symbolized abdication of will when it was a matter of me.

Holding my ground, I launched into my fear of addiction; that once I started on something, I'd use them for the wrong reasons, just as I had done with narcotics, cigarettes, and still did with alcohol and food. Dr. Kane was quick to refute a risk of addiction, either psycho-logically or physically. In order for something to be addictive, it must work quickly. Antidepressants do not, he informed me; in fact, I might not notice any change for three to four weeks. Hearing that, I could only wonder what one was expected to do in the meantime. Nevertheless, I remain unconvinced that dependence, if not addiction, was not a valid fear. While the drugs themselves may not be addictive biologically, the relief they offer may cause psychological dependence for those with an addictive personality.

As if momentarily abandoning his cause, Dr. Kane proposed what he referred to as the more "trite" approaches to my depression: take time off work to do things I enjoy: read a book, go to a matinee, even go away somewhere if I feel like it; solicit a second opinion; come back to see him in two to three weeks; or "just see how things go." With that, he scribbled his name on the bottom of an 8 ½" x 11" sheet of paper, ripped it off and handed it across the desk. Should I change my mind, I was to give him a call. "Forget it buddy," I thought as I stood to shake his hand and thank him for his time.

I left Dr. Kane's office in a daze. Out into the cold March air, down the stairs of ARF, standing still on the sidewalk; which way to turn? Intellectually, I understood and accepted the significant bio-logical component of my depression, but I had spent half my life self-medicating with contraband, alcohol, and food. Succumbing to anti-depressants represented to me a total failure and loss of control to yet another substance. As I had watched happen to Mom for the first 20 years of my life, I feared parts of me would be stolen that I would never retrieve. With the world closing in around me, I had no idea how I was going to get out. Turning to the right, I walked and walked for what seemed like hours, mentally preventing myself from being wrapped around the twiddling fingers of a shrink I'd never see again.

Twenty-six: Frozen moment

[MONDAY, MARCH 14, 1994] *I drag my weary body up the three flights of stairs, knock lightly on the door, and am greeted by the rich and comforting aroma of freshly brewed java. Taking my place on the edge of the couch, I can feel the pathetic desperation oozing out from beneath my chilled skin.*

VERY MUCH AT a crossroads, I steadfastly rejected the path of least resistance: one littered with cryptic prescriptions and pill-bottle warriors. The support for antidepressants was overwhelming, yea-sayers including Joan and Dr. Kane, my family doctor, many friends, and even my boss at that time, whom I felt obliged to update about my progress or lack thereof. She encouraged me to take the antidepressants, assuring me she would tell me if she noticed any negative change once I started back to work. I knew it was difficult for people to understand why I would not choose to take something that would probably make me feel better, especially those who had been there. But a scared, yet unwavering voice inside me refused to accept that medication was the way for me to go. I clung to the idea that there had to be other methods to try before — or if ever —yielding to medication. According to Dr. Kane, I suppose I opted for one of the more "trite" approaches and decided to take time off work. I was granted two weeks to decide the rest of my life. At least the pressure of it made it feel that way.

[MONDAY, MARCH 14, 1994, 3:50 P.M. — JOURNAL ENTRY] *Passing restless moments before my 4:00 counselling session. Staring listlessly out at the street. Questioning what the hell am I doing here? What am I doing in life in general? Three days shy of my 32nd birthday, I am stagnating in a progressive depression of some eight months, wrestling with the reason for my existence, struggling to keep the suicidal fate of 32-year-old Cree artist Benjamin Chee Chee from becoming my own. Days earlier, I'd been introduced to his artwork, and could not seem to get his tragic demise out of my head for no other reason than that he had only lived to the age I would soon be. A native of Temagami, Ontario, Chee Chee was driven to succeed as an artist. It was his dream that success would find him reunited with his mother, of whom he had lost track. I could relate to his quest, as metaphorically, I too had lost track of my mother over the years, dead as she was in throes of her depression. Tragically, Chee Chee chose death by his own hand before the maternal reunion could take place. My heart, however, was still somehow beating.*

During that fortnight in March, one of my strongest allies against medication was my counsellor Claire. I'll never forget Monday, March 14, 1994, as the day she asked me what I would do if I had only six months to live. My immediate response was that I knew what I wanted to have already done when I had only six months to live: write a book. Working on a book about our family's experience with depression had always been in the back of my mind as something I imagined myself doing, but at some distant age, with a career under my belt, and when financial security would give me licence to write under the shade of a tree by the side of a shimmering lake. But at the rate I was going, the odds of drowning before I'd reach the shore were more promising.

Before I left that day, Claire handed me a copy of Natalie Goldberg's *Writing Down the Bones*, aptly subtitled *Freeing the Writer Within*. She knew me well enough by then to know I would identify myself lurking between the covers of this wonderful book. In her foreword, Judith Guest, author of *Ordinary People*, the intensely emotional film of the same name I have been drawn to numerous times, referred to

Writing Down the Bones as a book that could even save a life. If the end of my life were as near as it felt, I would at least attempt to pay homage to the passion I'd long harboured. The flames danced seductively around me. To douse them was to die; to write was to live. It was in that Mortimer Avenue apartment, darkened by late afternoon shadows, that I experienced one of my frozen moments: those precious instants of enlightenment, so innocent, yet so powerful as they proceed to alter your life forever. Ninety minutes later, I departed, vaguely aware that a corner of the cloak of my doom had been lifted, revealing what at that time I clung to as the only reason to live: writing this book. I embraced it as the salvation that would somehow guide me out of the shrinking cave of my existence; away from the eerie image of a dead Cree artist whom I had never met. But where that image faded, another one burned ominously: that on the edge of 32, I was the same age my mother had been when she gave me birth. Something inside was luring me to admit that I'd come full circle.

The logistics of it all were almost secondary; namely, whether or not I was in a financial position to leave my job. Yunee, who was understandably at her wits' end with me, allowed that if quitting my job was what it would take to make me feel better, so be it. Although my income was important, we would manage on my savings and her income. Despite the instability of our relationship, she somehow trusted me to know what was the best decision for me. For what is the value of money when you are emotionally bankrupt? I felt like I was taking a huge leap off the edge of a cliff — no safety net below. But the alternative had exhausted itself. My shoulders gave out under the pressure of simply having to get up and go and juggle the multiple demands on my time. I admitted defeat. With no foreseeable end to the crushing heaviness of being, I could no longer fathom continuing to work.

When I shared my decision with Joan at ARF, she questioned whether it was not a rash decision, that my best option would have been a more conservative one to opt for a leave of absence. Yunee also later told me that she felt I had been coerced into the decision to leave my job. Granted, I was in a vulnerable and impressionable state at the time I made the decision to quit. Nevertheless, Claire guided me toward a vision that I embraced from my gut and my heart, if perhaps not my head: that it was possible to leave the security of a well-paying job and step into the fire of my dream and the light of my reason for being.

Once I had submitted a letter of intention to my boss, and when the call came from human resources to confirm my decision to leave, the words "official resignation day" struck me with an implosive finality. One of the skeletons in my closet ever since has been the guilt about leaving that job and the circumstances that precipitated my leaving. I very much felt as if I had failed the woman who had risked her credibility by promoting me so well for the position I ended up leaving 18 months later in a shameful mess. It was as if I was thrust back to a time so long ago, when the shame of my mother's sickness governed our lives.

I cried a bucket of tears when I cleaned my office out Easter Sunday, April 2, 1994. It was of little consolation that a colleague was there with me and kindly offered to drive me home with my things. She had been someone in whom I had confided, and at times I was aware of trespassing my vague emotional boundaries. Perhaps not so coincidentally, I have not spoken to her since. Ten days later, I met with my boss to hand over my keys and sign the paperwork. I felt like a leper daring to venture back into the healthy corporate arena. Making sure to arrive after the regular working hours, I anxiously awaited the elevator to whisk me up to the 18th floor, hoping I would see nobody familiar.

As fate would have it, the three colleagues I did see met my eyes hesitantly, their kind faces ridden with questions. I turned in shame and with tears stinging. What people understood, I do not really know. God knows I was not the only stressed-out person in the office, so why had I gone off the deep end? It was an alienating feeling to leave an office of some 50 people and a position through which I had contact with hundreds, with never a call or a note of concern afterwards from anyone.

During the months after I left that job, I had a phobia of being anywhere I might see someone related to work. Acute paranoia shadowed me, as on the afternoon in April when I attended a classical music concert at Roy Thompson Hall with Yunee and our neighbour Donna. My nervousness was an almost agoraphobic response to being in a crowd, and in such close proximity to my former place of work. The mood of the concert was spoiled, as I was unable to convey how panicked I was at the possibility of seeing a familiar face. When I did finally speak with a former colleague several months after I left, she admitted that she had been advised it was not a good idea to contact or write me. Hearing that her genuine efforts to offer support were sabotaged, in a sense reinforced my perception that people thought I was crazy. God knows I felt that way. I also thought back to what Mom must have felt like all those years ago, when depression kept her a virtual prisoner, suspended from social contact. I could not then handle Mom's depressions; I was fairing no better dealing with mine. I tried to embrace leaving paid work as running toward something, not away from. I was acknowledging what I really needed: to get off the roller coaster of life — or risk being crushed to death.

Once the decision to leave work was made, I then had to assess my home situation. When I committed to writing this book, my relationship of six years was in shambles. I felt I had to go somewhere to be alone, in order to sort out my life. I hated for Yunee to see me as I was, feeling pathetic and struggling to keep my head above water when in fact I was drowning and dragging her down with me. I questioned whether I could become better within the context of our relationship. But there was no room for grey in our world: once I left, there would be no coming back. I began to see how over the years we had been doing patch jobs each time our bond ripped open. As with my family, the wounds never healed, and now were exposed to the stale air.

We were eating away at each other. She deserved more consistency and fewer burdens in a relationship than I could offer. We were both all but resigned to splitting up; exhausted by the effort to continue the way we were. Yunee would buy me out. I would move out. The lawyer was called. The appointment made. There were no words for the heartache. There were no tears left to be cried.

And yet, the cold-blooded nature of what we were prepared to do, was, quite simply, too frightening. Hell as it had become to live together, it was inconceivable to live apart. We had invested too much to throw it away. An hour before setting a match to our joint tenancy arrangement, we reneged, granting ourselves an eleventh hour stay of execution. We dredged up more tears and trusted them to carry us along on a winding river of hope. Whether because of fear or faith, what we both had perceived to be irreparable damage was painstakingly salvaged. When I left my job a month later in April 1994, the anticipation of more shared time and probable confrontations peaked; incredibly, our relationship ameliorated exponentially. It was truly a season of renewal.

[APRIL 1994 — JOURNAL ENTRY] *Plethora of sights and sounds ...*
intoxicated by the nature around me ... mid-afternoon sun breathes gently upon my
bruised brain, my bulging body ... snowstorms of March past now seem so distant
... spring pleading with winter to bid adieu ... digesting the serenity of our home in
the woods ... the emotional burdens of winter melted, fertilizing the ground as
naturally as rice water penetrates the plants ... the glistening of the creek rushing
below, peeking through still-naked branches ... squirrels and birds and I rejoice in the
adorning buds of spring ... no more the stale crumpled leaves of fall ...

By the time I brought forth that piece of positive writing, I was experiencing stability unmatched in months. Headstrong into May with sights set on June, I would cautiously say I felt better, though my confidence and esteem were not yet fully restored. I still cowered in an almost Pavlovian manner in response to questions about the job I'd left.

During that newly embraced period of wellness, I took nothing for granted. I struggled with the idea that if I were able to get better without medication, had I really been clinically depressed? Was it all in my head? My readings and the ongoing counselling with Joan and Claire reinforced that medication is only one way to treat depression. Bypassing that road as I had is not an option for everyone. With Yunee's financial support and encouragement, I was granted the luxury of time to embark upon my own restoration process; to get back in touch with everything I had perhaps not really lost, only misplaced. The sights and sounds of that spring day in April offered reprieve from the chaos within. Had I not climbed off the rickety roller coaster of my life as it was and began shedding the old baggage, the ride would have most certainly ground to a halt, pinning me beneath the rails.

The months after leaving work were a process of re-learning how to take one step at a time, and of accepting that life for me is not defined by promotions, money, or greatness, but by small and often private victories. The reality of that is still reinforced each time I am downtown in the midst of the hustle and bustle, where time is money and the soul is so easily lost in the shuffle. Becoming more in tune with my own pace and trying not to compare myself with others who have seemingly rougher roads, yet who accomplish more, have been two of the biggest hurdles to overcome.

Even though I knew in my heart I was making the right choice to resign, I was worried about what my family, Yunee's family, some of my friends, the neighbours, even people I barely knew, would think. I feared Yunee's family would think I was living off her comfortable income. I was afraid the contingent of Protestant work-ethic neighbours would cast me off as a lazy bum. I dreaded the idea that those who knew about my Mom's past would assume I was following in her footsteps. For months, I refrained from telling my parents that I had left my job; I preferred to keep Dad's inquisitions and Mom's excessive worry at bay.

It was months before I started to accept that maybe it was okay, and I would allow myself to go out of the house, during the day when most people were "supposed" to be at work. For me, the writing *was* work, perhaps the most difficult I have ever done, for it necessitated that I take ownership of what was best for me.

When this book was still in the embryonic stages, Yunee and I spent a weekend with our friends Diane and Bob at their wonderful cottage in the Haliburton Highlands. It was one of those blissful late spring evenings drinking beer by the campfire, bonding with nature and each other, when I tried to explain what I was writing. Like an artist who tries to lend meaning to an unfinished canvas, my reason for writing was equally abstract. Though my head was full, the process was still raw and my confidence frail. My words sounded silly, and I found it easier to lose myself in the fire; perhaps one day the work would speak for itself.

time tunnels

the waves of wisdom
lap softly toward
the hollows of two
time tunnels
which both beckon
the wayward souls
who question through which
life's journey will be most gentle
the currents of destiny
whisper the way
unveiling the strong and vibrant undertow
of an oft-troubled inner spirit . . .

Part IV: Damaged roots

Twenty-seven: Father root:

muted love

"If children live with criticism,
　　　　They learn to condemn.
If children live with hostility,
　　　　They learn to fight.
If children live with ridicule,
　　　　They learn to be shy.
If children live with shame,
　　　　They learn to feel guilty."
[DOROTHY LAW NOLTE —
"Children Learn What They Live"]

QUITTING MY JOB in order to write paved the way for me to progress to a deeper level of introspection. As I became more entrenched in this book, it became clearer to me how damaged our family system had become. Beyond lack of communication, an unhealthy root system in our family of origin has prevented us from establishing and nurturing consistent bonds. The critical time to forge sound alliances was stolen by years ravaged by Mom's cycles of depression.

　　Her depression had stunted the growth of the individual branches of our family tree, dangerously depleting the nutrients for viable buds on branches to bloom. Depression remained an albatross around our necks, wearing thin our frayed and fragile family ties, magnifying the emotional voids between us. It is no more apparent than in my own inability to say, "I love you" to my parents and brother: years ago I had clipped out an Ann Landers column entitled "Don't Wait to Say I Love You." The paper, now yellowed with age, hangs on my bulletin board. Yet I still have enough fingers and toes to count how many times I recall having told them so. When I think in those terms, I am ashamed and seek to console myself. Surely when I was little I told my parents I loved them? All children do.

But as an adult, those words rest in the deep recesses of my heart every time I speak with Mom on the phone. At the end of our conversations, she unfailingly blows kisses through the mouthpiece. I reply with an awkward "thanks," not able to respond in kind, or tell her I love her, knowing it is the best gift of all I could give her. Perhaps vast emotional deserts were merely the destiny of our family. We existed only as names to each other, having long ago eroded the basis for a healthy communication among all limbs of a well-nurtured tree; roots seeking for, but never finding, fertile soil. The condition of the soil where my father is concerned is especially caked over from years of communication drought. Even when he underwent triple-bypass surgery in his late 60s, I could not utter those three little words in the few moments before he was doped up with anesthetic and whisked away; in spite of a little voice screaming inside that in the event of complications, I might never see him again. The years had taken their toll: I simply could not bring myself to utter those three words.

A seemingly trivial example captures the perennial deep-seated rift in the relationship with my Dad; a chasm born of his inability — or unwillingness — to really listen to what I have to say:

[JUNE 1994] Calling to let my parents know I'd be coming in for Father's Day — maybe they'd like to go out for dinner. As I spoke with Mom, Dad was yelling in the background for her to tell me to forget about Father's Day. Though I should be immune to his gruffness around such events, the familiar wave of discouragement washes over me. Nevertheless, I carried through with my plan to cycle to Hamilton, a journey of some three hours that I had often considered doing. If Dad were going to be in one of his ogre-like moods when I arrived, at least I would have the achievement of the ride to fall back upon and feel good about. Sure enough, from the time I arrived in mid-afternoon, until my departure the next morning, the mood was less than cheerful.

The climax came when Dad announced he would drive me down the mountain with my bike in the trunk; it would be safer that way, he informed me. Innocently enough, I thanked him, but said it was okay, I'd cycle down just as I'd come up. When he insisted, I knew immediately where we were headed. Dad was playing the wounded child and I was to appease him. My words rang hollow as I tried to explain how the challenge of riding up the mountain was balanced by the thrill of cycling down with the wind in my face, the city of Hamilton below me. But that day, I'd pushed him too far, and he had no interest in my rationale. Our parting was less than amiable.

As frequently happens, he donned his *"do-whatever-the-hell-you-want-to-do-I-don't-care/you-never-listen-to-me-anyway-so-what's-the-goddamn-point?"* attitude. His words cut into me in the still tender hours of the day. They suffocated me; reduced me to his version of a disobedient and disrespectful daughter. It's always a power struggle between us. Dad wants to do something for me; I prefer to be independent and make my way down alone. I am afraid of his anger, but refuse to compromise on things he knows I enjoy, like cycling, a means of physical and mental exercise for me. Dad perceives my refusal as shutting him out. I insist I appreciate his offer. But all he hears is the voice of an ungrateful daughter. We reach this proverbial impasse time and time again. The irony of it all is that the independence I was forced to acquire at an early age by virtue of my mother's illness is now perceived as "goddamned stubbornness."

I'd not planned to leave quite so early, but by 7:00 a.m. I had to get out. I bid a tearful good-bye to Mom as she watched helplessly from the porch. Though I had cycled down the mountain numerous times while living in Hamilton and knew how to strategically wait for the break in traffic before starting, that day, I was trembling, unable to shake the feeling that Dad had placed an omen on my ride home. How easy it was for him to get me riled up. I made my way safely, even arrived home in record time; propelled by anger and frustration, but drained of mental energy, brow-beaten by the tug-of-war that remains a central theme in our relationship.

From time to time, I reflect upon tentative in-roads forged with my Dad through lengthy letters exchanged during my European travel. But that break in communication was a flash in the pan. Dad's repeated anthem is that he doesn't know how to communicate with me. He's right: he doesn't. Try as I might to shirk responsibility for that, I am programmed to soak up his not-so-subtle blame. Conversations of a minute or two are barely tolerable; our stillborn conversations my punishment — or his — for the past.

Where did we go wrong? One day I was the shy little girl, frolicking with my brother in the white caps at Sauble Beach, chasing seagulls along the shore, worried that one day Dad would leave us, and in the meantime, fearing his temper and his frightening verbal and physical fights with Mom when she was sick. While Dad always ensured Barry and I were well dressed and fed as he took over the role of dual parenting time and again, clothes and food do not a lasting bond make.

As a teenager, a deep-seated resentment of his chronic anger surfaced, especially when he directed it toward Mom when she was down in the dumps, bedridden with depression. It made it difficult for me to be around him, and next to impossible for me to foster a healthy relationship with him. Over the years, we stagnated in the passive-aggressive rut of daughter and father. As an adult, groping for ways to make amends for our strained interaction, I foresee it will be the forfeited opportunities to appreciate each other as individuals that one day I'll live to regret.

unsung hero

with different eyes i see you
through photos which tell a story
from the small boy carefree by the cannon's side
his smile seems to encompass the bay
yet as the years crept by, i sense sadness mounted
though disguised so no others would see
a teenage boy and then a man
upon whose shoulders the world was carried
despite a severed father-bond
you yourself became a dad
not quite my age when i was born
your face glowed as you held me proud
yes, there was a time when the laughter flowed
and barriers were only to keep me from falling
but then, as destiny would have it
we became as two ships barely passing in the night
now a painful restoration — a struggle to wash the wounds
inspired by the scars themselves, and four decades full of memories
those moments captured through a father's lens
speak volumes eternally etched in my mind
the care you took for all of us, your sacrifices made
went often unpraised, though you toiled away
you did your best to give what you could
i wish those years could be somehow repaid
shrouded by gloomy clouds of grey
how sad it is
that but a trauma bond and blood
is what we have in common today...

Twenty-eight: Brother root:
castles in the sand

Between the rocks where weeds did ravage, the years were yanked right up; no holds barred, and words not minced, the sky came thundering down . . .

THE TURMOIL of the past drives a similar wedge between my brother and me. Only yesterday Barry was the blond-haired little boy with the mischievous grin, with whom I'd determinedly built empires of castles in the sand. How much those summers seem like another lifetime — and in a sense they were. A time when innocence was a virtue painstakingly tested, the worries of the world yet to be digested — or had they? For when the Lake Huron tide rolled in, destroying the finely molded fruits of our Sauble sand travails, we became adults before our time. The weight of childhood responsibilities was ours alone to manage. So many questions, fears and anxieties; not nearly enough answers.

[NOVEMBER 3, 1978 — JOURNAL ENTRY] *Barry is really pissed off at me. He was bugging me so I slapped him in the chest harder than I thought. I feel really sorry now. I really hate fighting with him. Felt especially awful when he said: "I don't like you very much anymore. You make me feel like a real scum." I always think about him getting depressed and killing himself. I hate thinking like that but it seems I do very often when he's not happy. I get worried about him too 'cause I want him to make good in the world and not be depressed about life. I guess all siblings go through this stage. One of these days, I know the fighting will end — at least when we're grown up . . .*

Barry and I struggled both together and separately to cope with our unstable home life. In our preteen years, I worried after him, for he was a scared and fragile little boy. At the age of nine, he stayed under his bed, threatening to run away for some reason. I recall being stunned that Dad was willing to let him go, not understanding the concept of reverse psychology at the time. All I knew was that without Barry, I was alone.

During high school, although our paths parted, they overlapped in the jungle of alcohol and drug indulgences. After Barry moved to Toronto in the early 1980s, on the surface, we went through a period of veiled openness, sharing guarded parts of ourselves when I stayed with him on weekend escapes. It was Barry, not my parents, in whom I had confided about a sexual assault in the early 1980s. It was I, not my parents, who knew about his clandestine relationships with girls and women. But over the years, we maintained a safe distance about our experiences growing up and how we had come into our own as adults.

It was one August afternoon in 1993 when the barricades collapsed, in the wake of a volcano erupting unannounced with a vengeance. One moment, we were landscaping in his backyard up in Port Perry; the next we were fisticuffs in his living room. Face to face with his rage, I was reduced to the terrorized sister he chased through the house when we were kids, threatening to beat me up. Had I followed through with my raised fist that day, as he callously taunted me to do, someone's blood would have spilled upon the plush carpet of grey. Though the skin remained unbroken, years of pent-up emotions were unleashed. Spitting up vicious words of criticism, he became my father, not the brother I'd cared for and worried about for so many years. But it was not those years in question. He was raking me over the coals for the most recent decade, when I'd been nothing but a vapour drifting in and out of his and my parents' lives. The deep-rooted anger in his voice was palpable, as if I had mortally wounded him. A torrent of blame was spewed at me, for shutting him and them out of my life. I couldn't help but wonder when we'd evolved into a family that demanded closeness.

Admittedly, I had progressively distanced myself over the years; told enough white lies to paint the wintry skies in the thickest clouds. As with Dad, any effort to explain myself to my brother fell on deaf ears. He had no patience for what he deemed my pathetic rationale; how I spent years hiding and lying, flushing my guts down the toilet, not to harm, but to protect them from the person I feared they'd despise.

In the wake of that summer day, everything backfired almost irretrievably. I was like a deer whose skittish gait entrapped her in her own vicious circle. Though the eyes beseeched mercy, time had run out. The rifle raised, the bloodletting imminent. The raw reality of our family dynamics was left like a bloody carcass upon the dry and brittle ground. Not to be diminished to a whimpering sister begging for reconciliation, I was a mere background presence at his 1994 wedding.

wedding bells toll

so proud am i, to have witnessed change
my little brother grown
you've reached beyond, to prove yourself
and found a path to please
but the sun does rise, to fall again
and with it, memories fade
the waters stirred beneath the bridge
have never quite been settled
briskly flowing, the current quick
with undertow uncertain
above those tides of turbulence
your wedding day will toll
washing away, upon the shore
the footprints silently cast
by an oft-forgotten distant wave
who despite all, remains your sister . . .

Twenty-nine: Daughter root:

for better for worse

"If you cannot find the truth right where you are, where do you expect to find it?"
[DOGEN ZENJI]

As THE turbulence in my family relationships can attest, the destructive and addictive nature of life past and present was in smouldering evidence all around me. Much to her credit, Yunee has been with me through the roughest times. Even when happiness in our relationship seemed irretrievable, the love somehow endured, and it was the very thread that allowed it to be repeatedly woven back together. I am eternally grateful for the force that brought us through such a violent storm. I could hardly have blamed Yunee if she had left me for good. I often knew that she stayed for the sake of C.C., our then-14-year-old Corgi-Terrier crossbreed, who was so attached and faithful to both of us. In many ways, our relationship mirrored that of each of our respective parents, who stayed together for reasons of self-sacrifice: namely, their children. C.C. certainly seemed to be the only thing Yunee and I had in common during those most trying times in our first half decade together.

By about November 1994, seven months after I resigned from my job, I could feel a true momentum building. Things were going so well, it was hard to believe at times it was my life. The days flew by with renewed purpose and achievement. I was experiencing more contentment than I can ever recall — happiness somehow was always of limited duration. Experiencing the passage of seasons in the ravine behind our house was part of the restorative process. I had weaned myself off sessions with both Joan at ARF and Claire. The emotional stability in my life was evidently not a fluke. The depression was further at bay, and I gradually stopped looking over my shoulder, anticipating a resurgence. The real barometer of change was regaining my running rhythm through the fall and winter, with sights set on my second marathon in May 1995. As I rode the wave of wellness, I hungered to call friends, something I'd not been able to do for months without inciting their concern over the poorly camouflaged despair in my voice. I thought of Mom, and how phoning her friends had always been an indication that she had once again triumphed over another cycle of depression. Where had I been all my life?, I wondered as I picked up the phone. After years of being on the fringe of many friendships, it was a relief telling people I'd never felt better. How grateful I was for the circle of souls who, time after time, were there for me whenever I stepped back into the land of the living.

I'll never forget the words of Peigi, my friend since childhood: *"We just want you to be happy. We've been waiting for you to find your way ..."* She, along with my other friends Sharon, Elaine, Kim, Susan, Jenny, and Danielle, has known me since grade school, into adulthood, through years wrought with reckless episodes of "acting out" behaviour. They have waited, watched helplessly from the sidelines, just as Mom's longtime friends had done over the years of her depressions. Whenever I fail to understand the logic of their persistence, the words of Thoreau, inscribed on the small wooden plaque once given to me by my friend Kim remind me: *"All I can do for my friend is to be a friend ..."* What more can anyone ask?

Where there had been barely a flicker of hope Yunee and I would "survive to '95," as 1994 came to a close, we were enjoying the twinkling lights on the Christmas tree, the scent of pine around us, surrounded by decorations I thought I had boxed away for good one year previous, never again to find themselves shared between us. It was as if I was granted another chance to begin again — yet again.

In February 1995, I attended an emotionally charged forum on depression at the University of Toronto. Sponsored by the Clarke Institute of Psychiatry, the guest speakers were Helen Hutchinson, former *Canada A.M.* and *W5* broadcaster, and Mike Wallace, of the famed television news program *60 Minutes*. The hall was filled to capacity: all races, shapes, sizes, physical abilities, and both genders. Depression heeds no boundaries in the lives it affects. That evening, I heard very real people speak of the very real issues that had long been our family's closeted, and shameful, reality.

Each in their turn, Helen and Mike shared their ordeals with depression, united in their plea for support and encouragement for not only depressives themselves, but for their caregivers. As Helen Hutchinson implored, "depression is truly a rotten disease." It is one that permeates many lives, causes pain to others, and is "hell on kids" who live with depressed parents. It is an illness that remains sadly misunderstood by those who watch from the wings, goading the afflicted individual to "just snap out of it." It takes much more than that. And more than drugs. At the very least, it takes time, patience, forgiveness, understanding, and unconditional love, none of which can be bought or sold. Only then can the wheels of wellness be set in motion. "It takes one to know one," Mike Wallace stressed. His words also resonated within me, echoing Mom's laments over the years that nobody understood what she was going through. The tears slid down my cheeks, thinking of how Mom had walked down the long and winding, frightening road of debilitating depression virtually alone; that even I as her daughter had not understood then what I could now. I had failed her then and am convinced I continue to do so.

A particularly nasty aspect of depression is the way in which it sneaks up on you for no apparent reason. Such was the case in February 1995. Everything had been going reasonably well, most importantly my writing and my relationship with Yunee. Waking one Saturday morning, I was overcome with lethargy, and the panicky feeling that I did not want to get up and go to the weekly Korean class I had been attending since September. As the day progressed, I felt increasingly worse, bursting into tears, yet unable to pinpoint why. Although I was not very communicative, Yunee's mere presence was comforting. Before leaving for her evening shift at the hospital, she did her best to cheer me up. By late afternoon, alone in my misery, I felt lousy, and sought solace in the better portion of a two-litre ice-cream container. Such comfort is fleeting, of course; merely a quick fix followed by a crash that cast me into a junkie-like stupor. I remained at low ebb right through until mid-week, relieved to be unencumbered by a nine-to-five job with its demands of psychological clarity.

Tuesday, the anxiety of Yunee's appointment with a specialist regarding the nodule her family doctor had detected on her right breast was put to rest: it seemed to have disappeared. I think we both expected the worst, and the emotional release was intense. Over the next couple of days, the fog lifted and I was back to my "usual" self. Although I tried to pass off my downward dip as a combination of PMS, the specialist appointment, or merely the February blahs, deep down the powerful food–mood connection was crystallizing in a way I had never fully accepted. Though my bulimia was still in remission, the paradox of food as both comfort and mood-altering agent suggested that eating could also maintain and even fuel a pre-existing emotional slump. Although that cycle was short lived, it was significant enough to abort what had become my daily routine of writing, running, and housework. With the exception of that brief setback, 1995 was a fairly stable if not tide-turning year.

Without a doubt, a cornerstone of the year, and in fact of my life to that point, was in ever-so-fortuitously happening upon a notice posted at the Bloor-Gladstone Library in west-end Toronto, advertising the "Blue Pencil Room" program for non-fiction writers. Admittedly, I had only stopped into the branch to use the facilities before continuing my trek downtown. While adjusting my knapsack on the way out, I nonchalantly scanned the bulletin board in the front entranceway, when my eyes recognized the photo of esteemed author-activist June Callwood, who was the acting writer-in-residence for the program. Her role was to read and provide professional advice on manuscripts submitted and meet with participants to discuss their work. As I read through the description of the program, my heart was thumping, for the book I was working on seemed to fit the criteria. The December deadline for a maximum 20-page manuscript sample seemed reachable. Then I quickly came to my senses. The chances of actually meeting with this woman, an Order of Canada recipient, whose achievements as an author, journalist, and social activist I had long admired, were remote at best, considering the vast catchment area of each public library in the Metro system, where the flyer was posted for all to see. Nevertheless, with hands a-tremble, I boldly wrote down the necessary information, and established a time-line in my head; after all, what did I have to lose?

Running continued to be very much my salvation when the tide threatened to turn on me. With the support of my "coach" Yunee, I completed marathons in both May and October — a real coup, considering the shape I'd been in little over a year previous. Running grounded and liberated me in a way that is comprehensible only to those who share the same passion. By the end of the summer, Yunee and I even started a small home-based business making photograph greeting cards from the marvellous nature shots for which she has a remarkably keen eye. Through the fall and into the winter, I busied myself with writing, card sales, and general housekeeping. Certainly I had what some might consider the luxury of not working at a paying job. Not a day went by that I did not consider how fortunate I was to be free of monetary pressure at that point in my life.

Nevertheless, I wrestled with feelings of guilt about not contributing an income to the household. If anything, it was that thought process that intermittently cast a shadow over my mood. But I was my own worst enemy, for Yunee supported the decision to stay home entirely. We were comfortable financially, carried no debts, had money in the bank and in RSPs: how much more fortunate could we have been?

Incomprehensible to some, I felt like I was working harder than ever. Instead of swallowing myself up working 10- to 12-hour days to meet deadlines, chair meetings, organize conferences, write proposals, and God knows what else, I was working to get my life together — perhaps the most difficult job I had ever had. Instead of earning an income, I assumed the bulk of household responsibilities, even spending more time cooking and gardening, two domains that had been primarily Yunee's. By being more present in the relationship, I was also better able to provide her with emotional support, as she repeatedly fought to keep nursing-career burnout at bay.

On December 15, two hours before the 4:30 p.m. deadline, I submitted a portion of my manuscript to the "Blue Pencil Room." After doing so, I suddenly regretted I had mentioned it to friends and family. What a fool I'd been, daring to hope something would come of it. Nevertheless, it was a tremendous relief to feel that I had accomplished something that year. My pitcher was slowly filling, and there was even a glimmer of hope that the ongoing estrangement from my brother showed promise of resolution, when we both went to my parents' for Christmas, and spoke to one another, after more than two years of silence between us.

Thirty: Waves against the rock

Polar opposites of office walls. Blacks, greens and blues of the waves crashing against the rocks before me; juxtaposed with the pastels and purples of an inner harbour, basking in the still waters of sunset behind me . . .

THOUGH RECONCILIATION with Barry alleviated a huge family burden, the year 1996 rang in under a shroud of despondency. Between January and April, cycles of wretched gloom were recurring until the clouds refused to disperse. I found myself crying for no apparent reason other than inexplicable despair. I'd even run miles through my tears, for to stop running was to admit defeat. As lousy as I felt, I was even more distressed by the way my state of mind was affecting Yunee. Joined at the heart, we share a common artery through which emotions are so easily siphoned. It is hard for her to know what to say or do, when I tearfully tell her that nothing helps. I can only wait for this melancholic state to pass. What I need the most is for her not to be mad and just be with me, not lose faith in me — as I was quickly losing faith in myself.

The one bright spot during the first four months of 1996 was in meeting with June Callwood, the author to whom I had submitted my work back in December. I'd all but conceded that I must have been one of hundreds of aspiring writers vying for a limited number of appointments with her. Thus, it was quite a shock when I was notified at the end of January that my time slot had been arranged for March

5th: a mere six weeks away. My spirits lifted, I apprehensively waited the day, for seldom is one afforded such access to public figures in this day and age, certainly in a metropolis the size of Toronto. Meeting with the author that blustery March day was indeed an honour. Furthermore, the potential that she conveyed in my work far exceeded my expectations, and left me feeling I was one step closer to realizing an impossible dream. We agreed to keep in touch, with sights set on a September "deadline." Despite that privileged boost to my writing, I was bogged down by a nagging melancholy that had been nipping at my heels with disturbing frequency.

[MARCH 1996] A young high school teacher from Oakville, who had been missing for several days, is found dead in the Gatineau region of Quebec. Suffering from diabetes, she had long battled the reality of a life controlled by insulin. When she could stand it no longer, she headed to a chalet where she had found pleasure in her earlier years. When she was discovered, she was fully clothed, in a chair on the deck of the chalet she had never even entered. Such a tragic end to a youthful life, evoking discussions I'd had with Joan at ARF, about the parallels between antidepressants and insulin. I empathized with the young woman's powerful desire to be freed from an insulin prison; how it could be so intense as to perceive death as the only viable option. Were I ever to surrender my life to medication, I too fantasized how I might welcome the ultimate escape, as the only way to retain a sense of self; to stand up for what I believed in; to be never more a pawn in the psychological games of war in my life.

[APRIL 6, 1996 — JOURNAL ENTRY] *I desperately seek to harness the restorative power of warm water rushing over me. To cleanse this precarious mood. Inhabited by the foreboding feeling there is a clouded entity mocking me overhead. Through my tears I see Mom and wonder, was it always this way for her?*

If I ever failed to legitimize the extent to which verbal assaults were a common occurrence growing up in my parents' home, Easter Sunday, 1996 shoved the grim truth down my throat yet again. As per usual, Dad was on Mom's back about still having to refer to the cooking instructions on the bag of frozen green beans. On one hand, his ranting and raving is anger inducing, an emotion I am both consciously and unconsciously aware of smothering. On the other, I regard his outbursts as pathetic attempts of his wounded child screaming to get out. It is a tragedy that he has not resolved issues that arose long before Mom was sick. Now she is better, he still feels he can verbally abuse her, as if exacting revenge for his sacrifice to stay with and support our family. I abhor the way he treats her. I see her wither like a wounded puppy and I want desperately to make up for that. But there is no room to navigate around the huge chip on his shoulder.

That day, he was on the warpath and also zeroed in on Yunee as his target. Her innocent attempt at discussion erupted when he yelled that she wasn't listening to him. I was ashamed and furious. It's one thing to talk to Mom and me like that. It is totally unacceptable to treat a guest in a similar manner. My urge to overturn the dining-room table in one fell swoop of rage was only quelled by Yunee's quick eye movement, signalling me to stay calm. Choking back anger as I had always done, we left the stone-cold silence of my parents as soon as we could when the dishes were done. Mom was like a lost puppy, caught in the middle.

My anger climaxed the next day with the first bulimic relapse in over a year. How I hate what my father's controlled domination does to me. How I hate what I do to myself.

[APRIL 8, 1996 — JOURNAL ENTRY] *Scrubbing myself raw in a shower as hot as I can stand, crying in shame, embarrassment, sadness, fear, and anger, for the cyclical nature of it all. Broken blood vessels betray my deed. A beer so cold it cuts a*

crystal clear path down my parched, ragged throat. I am consoled by nothing. I have
failed myself in shovelling rage, setting fire to the burnt out shell of my soul . . .

Days later, when I spoke to Dad, there was not one iota of remorse; there never has been. It is always the one on the receiving end of his rage who suffers the lingering effects: the depression of anger always backfires.

[APRIL 12, 1996] Phone rings. It's Dad. Calls to thank me for the birthday card I'd dutifully forced myself to send him. Tells me I sound as lousy as I did six months ago. Just not feeling good that's all, I mumble. He's angry that I have not called the doctor yet; that I am still not taking any medication. "What would have happened if your mother had not taken pills?" he challenged. I refrain from callously retorting that we'd probably be visiting her grave. He refuses to speak to me when I have only monosyllabic answers. "This is stupid," he barks and switches the phone over to Mom. I am numb when he speaks to me like that, instilling a defiance to stand my ground. Mom is clearly worried. She nearly pleads with me to take pills if the doctor offers, for her sake. She has never said anything to me as overtly persuasive as that before. I feel guilty for not doing what she asks. Part of me is tempted to go against my principles and take some damned drugs; to make her happy, just so she won't worry about me. I wax and wane and feel I'm going insane. I also fear that Mom's concern for me will trigger the end of her 14-year remission.

Running through the ravine behind our house, I can think of nothing else for days. Like the squirrel scurrying along the path with the coveted nut do I run, seeking to salvage myself. I decide to write my parents a long letter, in which I try to explain my personal reasons against medication. "While I do not dispute that lithium has been a 'miracle drug' for Mom, our situations are different. Mom does not have a choice; but I think I do. I believe I am making the right decision by not wanting to take pharmaceuticals. It means that I have to try my damnedest to alter my chemical composition in other ways, like watching what I eat and drink, exercising daily, writing, and leading a life as stress free as possible." Admittedly, I knew I didn't have much of a case as far as they were concerned, for whatever I was trying to do, obviously wasn't working. And no defense holds water in those juryless trials by Dad.

By May, I was virtually agoraphobic, most days shutting myself off from the world when Yunee left for work each afternoon. I would not answer the phone, kept the doors closed on even the most beautiful of spring days, and waited to walk our dog C.C. after dark. I struggled to write through the down times, waiting for an opportunity when the wave would eventually recede. As I continued to refuse medication, the waves lingered perhaps longer than necessary. As fate would have it, the window remained firmly closed for the better part of May and June and the possibility of a September manuscript deadline was quickly eroding.

[MAY 22, 1996] After weeks of procrastination, I finally made an appointment with Dr. Michelle Jerome, the family doctor I'd switched to several years prior, after Dr. Wong prescribed Imipramine. Arriving at her office at Women's College Hospital, I was informed she had called in sick. Did I want to see the attending practitioner? After waiting nearly an hour, I explained my symptoms to the kindly, if rushed, on-call doctor. Her eyes bore through me in a sympathetic way as my tears poured out. I was ashamed in my vulnerability. Her advice was antidepressants and to book an appointment as soon as possible with my regular doctor. She also recommended sessions with a psychiatrist, whose name she gave and offered to get back to me with the number. She never did get back to me, or return my follow-up call. After all, I wasn't her patient.

[MAY 29, 1996] When I met with Dr. Jerome the following week, she agreed with her colleague and recommended antidepressants. Though I'd been through my reasons against medication before, she assured me there were "some good ones out there now." I asked her about alternatives, to which she provided me with the names of four psychiatrists. By the way, she was leaving, she mentioned as I rose to leave. My file would be transferred to another doctor on the team. I left that day with a scrap of paper and wishes of good luck. I was, in fact, nobody's patient. Just like Mom had been nobody's patient nearly 14 years before me. Tick, tick, tick, went the time bomb in my head.

Faced with the daunting task of finding both a new family doctor and a therapist of some sort, once back home, I pulled out the list of names Dr. Jerome had given me. With stomach juices pumping and uncertain of what words would come out of my mouth, I dialled the first set of seven numbers. My anxiety proved to be little more than wasted energy. The first three doctors had answering machines that informed callers they were not accepting new patients. The voice on the fourth machine was far from inviting enough for me to leave my name. Deflated, I set about trying to find someone on my own. Despite the depths I had reached, I salvaged enough concentration to source out potential avenues. The challenge was to identify which route I wanted — and needed — to go in. First and foremost, I wanted to work with a gay-positive female with sound knowledge of depression and addictions. Though my previous counsellor, Claire, had fit the bill two years ago, I recognized the need for someone with more medical expertise. I also needed to find someone who was covered under OHIP, which narrowed things down considerably. Even though I was eligible under Yunee's workplace benefits, there were restrictions on the number of visits to licensed psychologists or psychiatrists per calendar year. What if I needed more than a few sessions? How could I justify forking over something in the neighbourhood of a hundred dollars per week for therapy? Now, however, I believe that money is irrelevant when health is at stake.

Over the next couple of days, I scoured lesbian and gay community newspapers, directories, and a women's referral and resource group, even the yellow pages, for someone who fit my criteria. With each phone call, I hated the pathetic sound of my low, droning voice as I fought back the tears. Though many of the women I spoke with had experience working with depression and addiction issues, most were private counsellors, social workers, or unlicensed psychologists. It was like looking for a needle in a haystack to find someone who was both covered under OHIP and accepting new patients. Call after call, my list of possible options dwindled. The closest I came was a referral to a Dr. Judith Cove, a psychiatrist who, while not accepting new patients, offered to notify me if something came available.

Though she provided a glimmer of hope, my need was more immediate. I kept on with my search. The more calls I made, the more disheartened and panicked I was. What if I couldn't find anybody? All I really needed was for someone to explain to me why I was feeling the way I was feeling, and perhaps make some sense of the patterns in my life. As a last resort, I contacted the Women's Therapy Clinic at the Clarke Institute. A sympathetic woman regretfully informed me there was at least a three-month waiting period for an initial assessment. Similarly, a local municipal mental health centre in Etobicoke could not offer me an appointment until August. I accepted and was placed on their cancellation list. In the midst of my frantic phantom psychiatrist pursuit, Dr. Cove called back with an opening in her schedule if I was still interested. The glimmer of hope brightened.

[JUNE 5, 1996] Cycling an hour and a half across town on a gray and humid day, I arrived at Dr. Cove's office flustered and sweaty. Locking my bike to a post at the corner, I turned and made my way toward the building just north of St. Clair, stopping cold in my tracks when I saw her name on the directory facing Yonge Street: Dr. J. Cove, *Psychiatrist*. Blood draining from my face, I ran up the stairs as if passersby were snickering knowingly of my destination. What on earth was I doing? I had no idea what to expect other than the worst, whatever that was, when I walked through the door to her suite, certain my heart would burst out of my throat, so suddenly nervous I was to meet her.

A flood of first impressions washed over me. A quick glance around the small, tastefully decorated waiting room was interrupted by a surprisingly young woman who came out to greet me. As best I could, I tried to compose myself while she led me through to her office, convinced she could hear the adrenaline pounding through my body. Moving toward the seat she offered, as she quietly closed the door behind her, I shyly apologized for my sweaty appearance, while taking in her coolly clad person in fresh cottons of navy and white. For the next 50 minutes, I responded to her questions about the way I was feeling, my family history, and life in general. Was I suicidal? she asked at one point. Though I had never plotted out a specific plan, I admitted to frequently fast forwarding to a time I would no longer be here. But for the sake of my partner and my mother, I would probably never do it, I felt obligated to assure her, wondering what the hell she was hearing between the lines.

Her soft-spoken voice melted through me as I tried to absorb as much as I could: office conservatively eclectic; photographs of boats at sunset, evoking an east-coast fishing village; an impressive shelf of books; framed diplomas on the wall; a solitary floor plant; a tabletop watering pitcher; two paper tulips of burnt orange and banana yellow; a small gold clock on a neat, though not obsessively organized, desk; a soapstone carving of a kayaking Eskimo; a curious round window-like object, perhaps a porthole rescued from a long abandoned mariner's vessel; a finely woven Persian rug of burgundy beneath my well-worn sandalled feet; her sensible, navy leather sandals and an Indian cotton vest I would have chosen for myself. And behind her that dramatic David Blackwood print of furious waves crashing against a vast expanse of Newfoundland rock.

By the end of the session, I'd reduced myself to tears, and was aware of a stirring connection I was not sure I could handle. We agreed on another appointment for the following Friday. Rising to shake her hand, I thanked her for her time. Nine days and counting. Would I have the nerve to come back?

In the days that followed, I continued to investigate my therapy options, somewhat leery about staying with the first person I'd met. Before my next session with Dr. Cove, I decided to follow up on a referral to Jan Hiller, a lesbian psychologist referred by the Women's Resource Centre. By the time I cycled down to her office, I'd been caught in an absolute downpour. I sure wasn't having any luck with my arrivals at these appointments. As I was soaked to the bone, she offered me a garbage bag to sit on during the 90 minutes we talked. Her office was more like a university dorm room, with a futon mattress and pillows on the floor, candles, books, and posters everywhere. We talked and I cried, as if drawn into the spell of this Wiccan-like lair. As comfortable as I was with her laid-back style, my rational mind told me I needed to pursue a more traditional, medically oriented path.

My search for a new family doctor led me to Dr. Elsa Vander, a physician recommended years prior by my friend Pam. During my first appointment, Dr. Vander listened with reasonable compassion to my present state of affairs. In her trademark no-nonsense manner, she advised anti-depressants and a psychiatrist to get me back among the land of the living. Before I left, she scrutinized my tear-stained face, flashed me a cheek-to-cheek smile, and pointed out that the sun was shining: in other words, life couldn't be that bad could it? Cycling home with a fresh list of psychiatrists and psychologists, I noticed that the sun was indeed shining. Once home, I took a cursory look at the names on the list Dr. Vander had given me. As my eyes moved down to the bottom of the page, they came to rest on Dr. Judith Cove's. As fate would have it, none of the other names I called on Dr. Vander's list was appropriate for one reason or another. Something in the back of my head was telling me I'd already found who I was looking for. However skeptical I had previously been about psychiatrists, I recognized the need to pursue this avenue at that point in my life. I was compelled to go back to Dr. Cove, for I was one beggar who could hardly afford to be a chooser.

Over the course of the next three sessions, I revealed a little bit more about why I thought I was in her office. Dr. Cove ordered blood work to ensure that there was not a pre-existing physical problem, such as hypothyroidism or serum ferritin deficiency, contributing to the way I was feeling. We also discussed at length my nutritional habits, previous eating disorder, and substance abuse. When the assessment phase was complete, Dr. Cove's diagnosis was indeed one of clinical depression. For some reason, hearing that was a shock. Much as I knew how despairingly I had been feeling, it was still hard for me to accept that I was clinically depressed, for the image of depression in my mind has always been of Mom, staying in bed for days and weeks on end. I was not that bad. On the other hand, I was bluer than blue.

Dr. Cove heard me out. "You are not your mother," she gently, yet firmly, assured me, and went on to explain that depression covers a whole spectrum of symptoms and severity. Where my Mom had been at the extreme end, my experience was quite different. She cited the genetic predisposition and probable biological basis for my recurring depression. She also pointed out that depression usually occurs in conjunction with certain psychological factors. Her approach was to treat depression with a combination of pharmacology and psychotherapy. Faced with yet another doctor recommending antidepressants, I felt trapped. I knew medication could work. I understood that medications were more sophisticated now, and that ones in the SSRI family had fewer side-effects than the more traditional tricyclics, because they worked specifically on the neurotransmitter serotonin. Was I being too foolishly stubborn for my own good? Dr. Cove listened to my reasons against drugs, offered the logical rebuttals, but ultimately respected my choice, making it clear that the option was always there for me. I was surprised, yet relieved, that she was not giving me an ultimatum; that medication was not a condition of my ongoing work with her. It was important that she did not patronize me into changing my mind. To the contrary, she instilled in me the feeling that perhaps I was making the best decision for myself. That she demonstrated such trust in me was an early indication of how the framework of our sessions would progress.

When the formal process of psychotherapy began, I cannot be sure. Perhaps it was when Dr. Cove stopped writing and initiating the conversation, and began waiting for me to talk. In any case, I was too timid to ask whether what we were doing for 50 minutes was now psychotherapy. There was no mutual conversation like that I had been accustomed to with Claire. Rather, the sessions were a throwback to my therapy with Morgan at McMaster in 1985, when the silence between us had often been deafening. Eleven years later, I sat in muted awkwardness opposite this woman who evoked a sea of self-consciousness within me. I had so long depended on writing as a release for my feelings and emotions, that to disclose the innermost aspects of myself rendered me near catatonic before her. I'd read enough to know that psychotherapy requires a significant amount of work on the patient's side, so by the very nature of its structure, it was not going to be an easy process for a verbally inept individual like myself. The onus was on me to compose the agenda.

Despite the "homework" I'd do before each session, reviewing my notes from the previous week, my recent journal entries, and crib notes for what I'd planned to talk about, as soon as I walked through the door of her office, I was blank. As Dr. Cove would frequently point out, there were reasons for the anxiety, the silence, the closing myself off. Perhaps I had yet to develop more trust, she suggested. Though it had never occurred to me that I didn't trust her, her comment lead me to re-evaluate my definition of trust. I realized it was more an issue of not trusting myself to fully disrobe my feelings and emotions before her. But if I didn't talk, I was defeating the purpose of being there in the first place: to understand why I kept experiencing periods of depression and why this phase in particular was lingering so long. By then, it had been five consecutive weeks.

In some, depression is a warning sign of a growing external or internal stressor, such as relationships or a job. In short, it is the body's way of saying there is a problem. Cognitive-therapy advocates believe talking can change brain chemistry as effectively as medication, with results that are more permanent. By exploring and being more aware of how attitudes, beliefs, expectations, and thoughts can produce and maintain depression, it becomes easier to recognize distorted thinking patterns that damage self-esteem, create anxiety, alter such brain chemicals as serotonin, and thereby reinforce depression. The key in my case was to identify the psychological issues influencing my life and triggering the depressive episodes. When Dr. Cove initially asked me about things that could be bothering me, nothing out of the ordinary came to mind — at least not significant enough to warrant the way I was feeling. Things that had been factors in the past, such as my relationship and my job, were not problematic at that time.

Over the next few weeks, I did my best to open up to her. Gradually, I was aware that the fog in my head was lifting ever so slightly. With a tiny window of clarity cracked open, I began to dwell on the fact that I was editing out a significant part of myself: I remained closeted to her about my sexuality, and had an unnerving tendency to talk in riddles. By the tenth session, broaching the subject of my sexuality was unavoidable. Yet rather than directly telling her that I was gay, I cautiously explained that though finding a gay-positive psychiatrist had been a priority, I had not had the courage to address it when we first spoke over the phone. I braced myself for indications of her discomfort — my ticket to leave and never come back.

"I don't know what I can say or do to help you feel this is a safe environment. It's something you have to feel for yourself." In the same roundabout way I disclosed my sexuality, did she respond in her own indirect manner. Though relieved and reassured by her words, I wondered how the dynamics would shift, as I felt the old familiar angst beat butterfly wings within. How often I wished I could take flight on their frail appendages in search of safety in the face of vulnerability.

Ultimately, that unburdening was paramount to establishing an elevated level of comfort with Dr. Cove, and I was finally able to move ahead. Hearing myself speak, I began to visualize the link between thoughts and mood and how susceptible I was to negative thought processes. Dr. Cove's carefully worded feedback and perspectives heightened my awareness beyond a conscious level. But the anxiety of walking through her door week after week was at times paralyzing, despite her assurances that she was not there to judge me; there was no pressure to perform. Yet I was programmed to impress her, and to be deemed worthy of her time.

In part, it was my habitual way to overcompensate for being gay around people who may not be. Yet the precedence for my nervousness had been first established with Mrs. Michaels back in high school. The parallels frequently kept me from making eye contact with Dr. Cove throughout much of each session. I preferred the safety of the sky. I searched for the right words in the trees that swayed gently outside her window, or in the swirling waters in the painting that hung symbolically behind her. Whenever my eyes would shift shyly back to hers, I was certain my blushed cheeks betrayed what I was feeling, yet again.

Opponents of cognitive therapy believe you can talk for ages and feel even worse. Some sessions, I definitely left more disturbed than when I arrived, frustrated that I'd been talking in circles, wasting her time and nearly putting her to sleep. I was particularly uncomfortable when things I said about myself were linked with having a mother who had been ill during my formative years. It was too Freudian for me to accept, and I shut myself off from pursuing those angles with her.

I'd arrive home feeling raw and vulnerable, eating to fill an expanding crevice of emptiness and, at times, unable to resist the urge to drink. When I addressed the alcohol issue after one particular session, Dr. Cove cautioned that if therapy triggered destructive behaviour, then we needed to discuss why and perhaps reassess the decision to continue. Despite the qualms I had about the process of psychotherapy, I was committed to working through whatever was there. Quitting was not an option. I had already run from too many things in my life. There was a reason I was seeing a psychiatrist, and that I had been led to Dr. Cove's office in particular. In my heart of hearts, I knew I had barely scraped the surface.

Thirty-one: Layers of an onion skin

"I came here to find myself ... it's so easy to get lost in the world."
[Saugeen Indian passage, Southampton, 1996]

[JULY 1996] After weeks of relative isolation and seclusion, C.C. and I go for an early evening walk in the ravine. I feel in awe over the beauty of our "backyard" and cannot believe that I have been so out of touch for so long. Overflowing with need to feel the breeze and the sun on my body, I want to cherish this time so I will never again succumb to the drowning feeling of one trapped within the confines of self ...

As the summer progressed, I cautiously began to notice that my window upon the world was opening wider. My writing was coming more easily, my running was more fluid and a fall marathon seemed a possibility. I questioned the need to keep seeing Dr. Cove, for the depression had seemingly dispersed. Therein nestled the fallacy of my thinking. Dealing with the symptoms of depression was only part of the problem; the fact that I was no longer experiencing them did not mean I was "cured." I even naively wondered whether I had really been depressed, if I had been able to get better without medication. As Dr. Cove explained, the depression had merely exhausted itself. Given the cyclical nature of my depressive episodes over the years, it would most likely recur because I had not reached an understanding of the psychological issues that were festering within.

Sure enough, by November, mere days after completing a marathon in Niagara Falls and spending a few days at the Haliburton cottage of our friends Diane and Bob, I was sucked back in the midst of the vac-uumous fog. Passive suicidal thoughts once again crowded my days: roughly translated from Korean, I felt like I was "wasting the rice." Self-flagellation reached new heights, affecting my relationship with Yunee more than ever before. I began to not only hear, but also listen to the pathetic tone of my voice. When so down on oneself, respect in a relationship is not easily commanded. To exacerbate matters, a bulimic relapse and drinking binge in mid-November led me back to ARF, as an adjunctive therapy encouraged by Dr. Cove. I was assessed once again and assigned to a new counsellor, Christine Clarke, in the "Structured Relapse Prevention Program." I was ashamed and afraid to be returning for help. What the hell had gone wrong?

Dr. Cove stated frankly that she would be remiss in not recom-mending a course of antidepressants. At that point, I admitted to a shift in my thinking; to a large extent, for the sake of my relation-ship with Yunee. Much as I tried to deny it, a major trigger was the small business Yunee and I had started a year and a half previous. My plan had been to start the Christmas sales after the marathon, but as October came to a close and November arrived, I became more anxious, preoccupied with how I was letting Yunee down. I was scared by the way my moods were playing such havoc on my life. It was the classic chicken-or-the-egg dynamic: Was I depressed because I was not pulling my weight, or was I not pulling my weight because I was depressed? Perhaps if I did try antidepressants, I would be better able to handle the business anxiety. I valued Dr. Cove's opinion enough to reconsider my position on medication.

But again I stepped back from taking the plunge. Once I made the leap, I imagined losing myself forever. It must have been infinitely frustrating for those who knew I was refusing potentially helpful medication. I was clinging to the now threadbare theory that I could keep relapses at bay, though I could see how thin that defense was wearing. Much as I understood how drugs rebalance neurotransmitters, I stubbornly refused to risk them masking thoughts and feelings. I wanted to live through and deal with them, bull-headed as that was; to let the depression run its course, and deal with moods as they arose.

After a three-week cycle, the fog lifted and I was once again half-heartedly looking for a reason to stop therapy; after all, I wasn't sick. But as Dr. Cove would often remind me, "You don't need to be sick to be in therapy." It's more about understanding oneself, something that many can pass through life without doing.

Numerous times I have remembered those words, and kept up with our weekly sessions. With the symptoms of depression in check, I was in the position to burrow beneath the surface to where a whole sub-culture of issues simmered. Where I had imagined myself in the swirling waters below the cliff, now I had started to scratch my way up the sheer smoothness of the rock formation. Perhaps, as Dr. Cove suggested, also referring to the painting behind her, the serenity of the village on the other side of the cliff was my destination. Focusing on the dark, angry waters only kept me from naming what I needed: emotional peace. Those words were like a hot towel twisting inside me as I gritted my teeth to hold back the tears that betrayed my needi-ness. How I hated to admit her words made sense. In my heart and rational mind I knew she was right. Six months after walking through her door, I was ready to keep climbing, even if my well-worked fingers bled to the bone. There was no guarantee of a life preserver should I lose my grip and lunge back downwards, to be submerged yet again in the vicious sea of melancholy. It was all a matter of trust.

When I left work in March 1994, peace of mind was a vague memory. Mired in depression, I'd set out to retrieve a time when I had been set-tled within myself. As the months passed, I began to reach that plane of emotional peace — or at least so I'd thought. In retrospect, the place I arrived at was but a resting plateau, a place from which I could safely sit and survey the wreckage of the past, with a faint vision toward tomorrow. So secure I had been with my newly acquired peace of mind, I didn't notice when the status quo began wearing thin.

By 1996, the coveted perch beneath me began to crack. When the fog rolled in, accompanied by old familiar drinking and eating patterns, it was as if I had dug myself back into the original hole of destruction of nearly 20 years previous when I was a confused and wayward teenager. The task of digging myself out and moving beyond would be a daunting one. It meant chipping away at the solid mass of the past until it was reduced to small pocket-sized pieces.

As 1996 drew to a close, revisiting the teenage road to self-destruction was unavoidable, and I was at risk of repeating the same old cycles over and over again, until such time as physical death claimed me. I forced myself to read through journals I began keeping in 1978. A voyeur into my own life, it was clear how much remained unresolved, as the waves of emotion screamed out from the page. Instead of madly scrambling to pick up the pieces, applying razor thin Band-Aids to well-weathered wounds, a methodical analysis of the past was in order. With an actively passive audience present in the body of Dr. Cove, all that was missing was me.

I fought many times to be anywhere but present with her. But there before her, beneath the jaded memories, I cowered in my neediness. It was the shame of needing to talk about what I had only ever dared to visit in the diaries I was terrified someone would find. I had sabotaged that need long enough, dismissing the past and the urge to break free of it as silly and frivolous. After all, I'd never been physically or sexually abused by a family member; my relatives had never suffered crimes against humanity. Time and again, through many unsettling silences during our sessions, I berated myself for clamming up, not trusting myself to be fully open before her. I hated the way I edited the hell out of thoughts that raced like highways through my head, only to grind to a screeching halt against the tightly pursed lips of my mouth.

I was tiring myself, yet Dr. Cove's patience seemed limitless, as she sat waiting for me to connect with the loose threads of the past so knotted in my head. Arresting my fears and anxieties, I began to strip down, peeling off the layers of my onion-skinned life. And between the layers of depressive cycles and substance abuse, was nestled the matrix of self I hungered to claim.

Thirty-two: Mother root:

constant craving

Six months into sessions with Dr. Cove, it happened:

[November, 1996 — journal entry] *Walking my dog C.C. through the ravine behind our house, the mirage appears dancing seductively before me. Tears of enlightenment crystallize on my windblown cheeks as I listen to what the apparition whispers as she flits in amongst the trees, swaying in time to their eerily creaking branches. I walk alongside myself, an adult who remains a prisoner of childhood longings and teenage addictions, in an attempt to satisfy an almost constant craving for a nurturing female spirit. In my quest for that nurturing, I am inundated by more Freudian connotations than I can bear. But this spirit who surrounds yet eludes me is not daunted. She dangles a fine silken thread just out of my grasp, tempting, as always, my need to connect. I reach out between the virgin snowflakes, and grab hold of temptation. In an instant I discover who she is, in all of her many guises. She is the muse of a poem, the seed of a crush, the fleeting eye contact, the embodiment of those certain women whose paths cross mine. She is the mother who gave me birth, only to vanish thereafter. Making my way through the stillness of the woods, I instinctively know where to begin looking for her . . .*

Part of me doesn't know how I had the gall to uproot the seeds once the idea poked through the soil. Between the covers of my journals, there emerged common thoughts and feelings that haunted my psyche. Seemingly out of the blue, I threw caution to the wind and confronted those feelings by locating Helen Michaels, my former high school English teacher. In the late 1970s, she represented everything that I feared and desired, that I lacked and that I craved, that I still carried with me unresolved. On the pretense of soliciting her assistance as a reader for this book, I rekindled that past when I met with her in mid-December 1996. The days and hours between my initial phone call and our subsequent rendezvous were unnervingly restless for me.

I was afraid I would embrace my destructive drinking patterns in an effort to smother the feelings that were resurfacing with a vengeance. My new counsellor at ARF, Christine, cautioned against meeting with someone who triggered such intense emotion within me. "You don't need to go through the fire," she advised. "Could you not find someone else to be a reader for your book?" While her concern was valid, my short answer to her was "no." The long answer was far too complex. I was determined to go through the fire. It was the only way for me to make it over the bridge and toward the door I was com-pelled to re-open — a door that was opened for me many years ago, and behind which rested the source of a significant and symbolic undercurrent in my life. There was no relinquishing my hold of the delicate thread now. I was prepared to trace it back to the time when a shy adolescent was drawn towards someone who represented more than grammar rules.

I suppose I could well have kept the nature of the attraction safely in the past, had it not proceeded to shape me as an adult, in the way that I repeatedly connect with certain women at a deeper and more meaningful level than I had the capacity or maturity to understand as a teenager. The need to embrace that significance began to take on a life of its own. Though some things are better left unsaid, what you cannot communicate will run your life. While I harboured enormous conflict about reopening this door of the past, it was almost as if I did not have a choice. It even occurred to me that perhaps the door had never even been closed, but rather left ajar. On a cold, damp December day, I followed the thread through the door and found myself in a place I had never left.

I arrived early at our arranged meeting place on the outskirts of Hamilton with plenty of time to gulp down two very strong cups of coffee. Admittedly, it was not the wisest beverage choice for taming the butterflies within, but at least I refrained from the beer I would have preferred. As the minutes ticked by, I tried to occupy myself by writing about how damn nervous I was, hoping like hell I was not making a blind and foolish mistake. After repeated glances out the window, I happened to look up just in time to catch sight of a woman hurrying through the parking lot. My stomach tightened. It was she. Moments later, she walked through the door. She seemed to recognize her former pupil immediately, and moved toward me. I stood to greet her, the colour rising to my face as if on command.

As we began our re-acquaintance, it was easily apparent why I had been drawn to this woman nearly 20 years previous. My nervousness slipped away, replaced by a comforting familiarity. It was as if I was somehow picking up where I had left off so many years ago.

Meeting with Mrs. Michaels unleashed a tide of emotion. As each wave washed over me, I was pulled toward the bridge leading me back to a fork in the road, when the conflict of striving to be a good daughter was challenged by a burgeoning sense of self that went against the grain of all things I knew to be "normal." The need to please my parents at all cost had always been in direct conflict with whatever I may have needed for myself. I had instinctively learned as a young child that Mom's needs necessitated a silencing of my own. Nevertheless, beneath the surface, some very basic needs existed. The need to be noticed and liked, the need to be listened to and accepted, the need for encouragement and praise; all became sources of shameful, rather than normal, neediness in my mind. Especially the need for affection.

On that mid-December afternoon, in the space of a mere two hours and over several more cups of coffee, I allowed myself to look across the table and into the eyes of the mirage from the ravine. I choked back the tears, my whole body recognizing that I was finally coming to terms with what I have always needed, but have fought to deny. With the safety mechanism of Dr. Cove in place, confronting those needs in meeting with Mrs. Michaels was critical to guiding me back further, to places I had never permitted myself to go.

My many moods assault me — leaving me along the way. A lost soul searching. And if I find, or when I find, my self, I know not from whence I came, other than from within her . . .

Freud frequently attributed depression to loss in childhood and irretractable guilt. Though not a loss in the physical sense as through death, the emotional loss of Mom had begun with her post-natal depression. Deprived of solid maternal nurturing, of someone to always be there, maybe even with a smile or a hug, a vast emptiness grew within me. The absence of such intangibles that most children take for granted a mother will provide had far-reaching repercussions into my adult life. For nearly 35 years, part of me sought to dismiss the weight of that loss. Certainly any time it was raised by Dr. Cove as a possible influence on my present, I squirmed uncomfortably in my seat, simultaneously blinking back tears and irritated by the subtext of it all.

In retrospect, I did not know how to handle the validation she was offering. Once I allowed myself to let go of the denial, it was crystal clear that the way I move through the world is largely governed by a severed mother-daughter connection. That early rupture gave way to my difficulty identifying acceptable emotional and physical boundaries with others, particularly older women.

In lieu of whatever Mom was unable to provide physically or emotionally, I subconsciously began searching elsewhere. It was in meeting Mrs. Michaels back in the tenth grade that I first became aware of my unsettling longing to establish female bonds. Even though I was accustomed to being the "seen-but-not-heard daughter" and the timid student cowering in the back of the classroom, this woman was not about to let me get away with feigning such invisibility. When I'd sensed that, I had craved her attention, in a way I had never wanted anything before. It was a powerful undertow that drove me to impress her. All the while, I'd flirted with danger, as losing weight became an obsession and drinking destructively was embraced as a desperate attempt to dilute the intensity of the emotions she kindled in me. The confusion was overwhelming, for I feared I was craving something beyond that which could safely be spoken. At times, the craving was all-consuming, and I could barely meet her eyes, for fear she would read my mind, and know immediately how needy I was. It was as if I'd been testing the waters with her, to see how far in I could wade before I'd be over my head. I have been treading water ever since.

Can a drunken fish swim through fire without singeing all scales?

In the two decades since high school, the unsettled waters still churn within me. How resilient the craving has been to the passage of time, as I remain so easily attracted to certain women. Even the fleeting eye-contact or the most casual of conversations will stir a familiar need deep inside. For it is those brief moments in time that acknowledge my existence, my worth, my need to be liked to a fault. How I still fear eye contact will betray my need for female affection. As it began in a classroom so very long ago, so it continues. By the shores of the Red Sea, on a morning commuter train, over drinks in a bar, in the office of a psychiatrist, merely walking my dog around the block; virtually everywhere, I am susceptible to the magnetism of the female aura.

The guilt and shame of my needs are no less painful at age 35 than they were at 16. Although I am still prone to smother my feelings with alcohol and/or food, at least I better understand them. In working with Dr. Cove, I have managed to process and even reconcile the nor-malcy of some of my needs. In so doing, I am more cognizant of how alcohol does not drown, but rather magnifies the intensity of unresolved shame and guilt. Drink after drink, emotional boundaries become fluid and the temptation to cross over uncharted physical bor-ders is heightened, at times with near immoral abandon. Although my logical mind now concedes there is no map, no way of navigating my way back to my mother through other women, I keep trying. Perhaps to stop would be like giving up on my mother. And I could never give up on the woman who gave me birth. Nor will I ever be able to make amends for the way my birth became her sadness.

Thirty-three: My mother, myself

"The relationship between a mother and daughter is comprised of a very deep understanding of and support for each other. It is based on an enormous amount of emotion and love. There is no other relationship in the world where two women are so much like one ..."

[SUSAN POLIS SCHUTZ — "To My Daughter, with Love"]

GROWING UP, I had no concept of cause and effect; I could not make Mom sick any more than I could make her better. When I was old enough to know that Mom had become depressed right after I was born, it instilled in me that I was at fault for her repeated cycles of illness. That omnipotent child who believes she can make people happy or sad, sick or healthy, becomes the adult with an uncanny perception of what people may be thinking or feeling, and is especially quick to feel guilty for things well beyond her control. I became accustomed to assuming unwarranted responsibilities, flogging myself with canes of "shoulds" and "sorries," to friends, family, my partner, neighbours, even my psychiatrist. "What are you sorry for?" Dr. Cove frequently asks. "For being born," I once heard myself answer with hollow finality.

As a rule, Dr. Cove's facial expressions rarely reveal what she may be thinking in response to what I say. I will never forget her look of dismay as those three words froze in time between us. In her pensively direct manner, Dr. Cove broke the news that Mom's depression was not my fault; that it would (probably) have happened anyway, and was

merely triggered by my birth. I felt lightheaded. It was like being vindicated for a cross of guilt I'd so long dragged around. Nevertheless,
though intellectually I understood, emotionally, I was not wholly
pacified. How then were two decades of Mom's clinical depression to
be accounted for? The link between my birth and the onset of Mom's
illness was too deeply ingrained for me to be absolved of the guilt so
easily. Although Mom now has many depression-free years behind
her, my guilt has accumulated in other areas. In the same way my birth
brought her heartache not happiness, do I continue to betray her. In
my relentless search for a nurturing female spirit, I am denying her the
role reserved only for a mother. It is a role she periodically expresses
guilt about not fulfilling when Barry and I were young. It is a role I
still yearn for her to step into — or do I? For often when she expresses maternal concern over my well-being, I flinch; I harbour resistance
to letting her into my life as much as she would like — and probably
needs — to be.

There is so much ground to retrace, getting back to where we started; to a time before either of us knew the true meaning of guilt. Back
before my own depressive cycles took hold, before I began sabotaging
my sense of self in a bottle. Back before I forfeited my childhood
needs in a vain attempt to make Mom better. Back before that first
electroconvulsive shock treatment surged through her brain. Back
before she was a young mother stuck with a colicky newborn. Back to
the womb, when she felt connected to me. A time when we were
bonded as one. A time when I was she and she was I. Only there
could we hope to come to terms with the bond that has never been
ours to salvage.

I thought back to July 1995, and a premeditated meeting with Mom to
talk about the writing of this book. By 7:00 a.m. it was already blister-
ing hot the morning I cycled into Hamilton, but the sunshine was
encouraging. I needed every ounce of reassurance to navigate the

uncharted waters of the past. We decided to visit a new waterfront park in the north end of the city. Although our destination was somewhat of a disappointment in terms of landscape, the goal was not so much the visual aesthetics, as the opportunity to talk outside of the house. We — at least I — needed to be in a neutral environment, not one riddled with unpleasant memories. We walked along in silence for a while, each in our own thoughts. Finally, we settled on a bench well away from throngs of children on a summer day-camp outing. We quietly sipped on cool drinks to satisfy our dry mouths; Mom's a side effect of the lithium, mine brought about by nerves.

Fearing I would lose the moment, I began talking about my own experience with depression over the years, lest it seem as if I was lapsing right into an unexpected inquisition of her past. Eventually, I took a deep breath and ventured, "What do you think caused your depressions?" my voice like a scream that echoed out across the bay. With a sideways glance I watched her from behind my sunglasses. The expression I detected on her face was one of genuine puzzlement. Her eyes seemingly fixed on a pleasure boat gently bobbing in the distance, she replied, "Gee, I don't know … I guess I was worried whether I was taking care of you kids okay."

I don't know what I expected to hear, but her response stunned me: could it really be that simple? Gazing out at the water, she continued ruefully, "Maybe I didn't try hard enough — after all, you did it." I knew she was referring to the fact that I had never taken antidepressant medication to deal with my depressions. I quickly reassured her that I knew that was not the case. I had always tried to understand that she could not help herself. In retrospect, her experiences with depression had been far more severe than mine. I've been fortunate enough to eventually come through periods of depression without medication. It was not to infer that she too should have been able to do likewise.

Mom often lamented that nobody understood what she was going through when in the depths of her depression. The little bit of ground covered on that July afternoon took me a few precious steps closer to the woman who had given me birth. As the afternoon sun beat down upon us, its rays intimately revealed my mother in a light I had never seen her. Much as our experiences have been different, I could now better understand what I could not as a child and what most who know her never will. I understood that at the very least, her depression was an ongoing expression of the overwhelming anxiety that she was not a good enough mother. Just as I often feel I am not a good enough daughter, partner, friend, neighbour, co-worker, sister, or patient. I understood that she tried so hard to get out of bed, that she was paralyzed by her own fear of failure. Just as I frequently doubt my abilities as a writer, a business partner, even as a volunteer. I understood why, in 1970, she had carefully clipped from the newspaper, a series of twelve excerpts from a book entitled *The Search for Serenity*.

Twenty-five years later, when I came upon the brittle and yellowed passages neatly tucked away in the bottom of her dresser drawer, I understood; I too have file cabinets full of clippings and bookshelves overflowing with introspective literature. I will always understand the fighting need to be released from the bondage of failure: to cradle the richness of self-worth and positive self-image, the very image I have been longing to hold — that of my mother, myself.

As far back as I can remember, people frequently remarked how much I resembled my Dad. I was never particularly fond of being reminded of that, since what little girl wants to look like a man? Although I have my maternal grandfather's dimple, it was always Barry who people thought had more of Mom's features. Shortly after the waterfront conversation with Mom, I bumped into a neighbour of my parents whom I had not seen in years. I was filled with indescribable pride when she exclaimed how much I am the image of my Mom. Admittedly, I also have some reservations about being too much like her. Whenever I feel as if I have stepped into my mother's well-trodden shoes of despair, Dr. Cove gently reminds me "You are not your mother." But in so many ways I am. We are reflections of each other: near mirror images.

mirror images

i am her
in my endless worrying
i am her in
my will to please others
i am her
in my sense of humour and wit
i am her
in my muted anger
i am her in my search for serenity . . .

Part V: Courage to come back

Thirty-four: Emergence

"We are all on the edge of destruction and we escape by the skin of our teeth, and when we come through on the other side, we find there is a meaning to life ..."

[ALBERT CAMUS]

THAT WE emerged intact as a family unit from the wrath of Mom's recurring depression can be very much attributed to the supportive friendships in our lives. Many of Mom's friends from her late teens and early twenties have stayed by her through the years of her illness. I recall her remarking once that she is surprised they did. It is a common worry we both share that people will just give up, not bothering to wait around for us to pull through again. A Richard Bach quotation on a poster once given to me by my friend Kim captures that wondrous gift of enduring friendship: *"Your friends will know you more in the first moment that you meet, than your acquaintances will know you in a thousand years."* Though our friends could never have fully understood our many moods and lapses from the world, they knew we would eventually come around and were there to catch us on the rebound. How blessed we have been. There is nothing more reassuring than being able to pick up the phone when you are back amongst the living and hear the voice of a long-cherished friend. Yet for all the ones who have stayed, it is the ones who left which are mourned with haunting frequency.

I still grieve the loss of a childhood friendship, as made evident by my friend Trisha's recurring presence in my dreams. Our friendship dates back to Mrs. Yoshida's 1967 kindergarten class at Buchanan Park Public School. We were tight-knit up until Grade 6, when street boundaries necessitated that we attend different senior public and high schools. When we were reunited in Grade 13, at Southmount Secondary School in the fall of 1980, we easily re-established our friendship. As young adults through McMaster University, our bond strengthened. Trisha and I understood the world together; we knew all the lyrics to Bruce Cockburn's songs.

But in the spring of 1988, during the time I was mired in a long stretch of post-European depression and increased substance abuse, her music left my world. When I had taken her up on her offer to housesit for her parents for the winter and early spring, in retrospect, I was in no condition to take on such a responsibility. When her parents arrived home unexpectedly in mid-May, I'd had no chance to clean house or replenish the food and alcohol I had consumed. For all intents and purposes, it appeared as if I had betrayed their trust and abused the privilege of taking care of their home. What I would not give to hear the familiar melody of Trisha's voice once again. That hollow longing renders the music of the faithful chorus of friends who have weathered the storms from childhood into adulthood all the more bittersweet. Sharon. Elaine. Kim. Peigi. Danielle. Susan. Jenny. You have all kept the beat when I was way out of tune.

There will always be sorrowful reminders of a past from which our family hardly escaped unscathed. I remember my longtime friends Sharon and Elaine remarking how comforting it had been to come upon Cootes Paradise, a marshland on the perimeter of Hamilton, following their month-long European trip in the early 1980s. For years, I recall only waves of nausea washing me each time the carp-filled water came into view each time I returned to Hamilton. In my mind, Cootes to the west of highway 403, with the imposing Cathedral to the east, represented the gates of hell into my hometown. The journey to my parents' Bendamere Avenue home was for a long time a gut-wrenching odyssey back to the familiar battleground. How the graffiti spray-painted on a wall heading up the James Street escarpment used to taunt me: IT'S NEVER TOO LATE TO HAVE A HAPPY CHILDHOOD. I guess you just have to sort through the sadness.

Back in the room of my childhood, a dish garden on the dresser conjures up memories of the umpteen hospital visits we made to see Mom. Although the paint is chipping off the decorative figurines and the multi-coloured gravel has faded, the cactuses thrive, defying the odds of survival as Mom did. The sweet-smell of the Avon bubble bath she still uses evokes visions of her finally drawing a bath after days or weeks in bed, to scrub away the dry, stale skin and work up a lather of shampoo in her straw-like matted hair. The well-worn leather wallet she made in the hospital that I keep on my desk. Photos on the bulletin board above my computer: Sauble sands and Hawaiian tropics; forced smiles of children; a grim-faced Dad and a sad-eyed Mom; my parents' wedding day in 1958. The Mom I never had a chance to know, at a time before depression stole her away.

I keep these and other mementos in a shrine-like arrangement around me, as tangible evidence of our past, for it is from whence we came that we are where we are. And we are but walking reminders of the many battles waged. I need look no further than the milky white, circular scars of the electrodes on Mom's temples, the indelible badges of courage she dares not to hide. The cold war years since 1982 have been marked by failed attempts to forge a treaty of peace among our family of four; to join forces that we might disentangle ourselves from the web of depression. After years of swimming against the current, of running from memories, feeling like an uninvited stranger in my own parents' home, these days, now I want to hold on to those same memories forever. I need to be empowered, not controlled by, or hide from, the past. I am consoled by the Voltairean theory that things happened for a reason. Our quest need not be to discover the elusive El Dorado, but to cultivate the garden we were given. Back to the womb I let myself be guided, to be born again with a fresh perspective of my family of origin; of the mother who brought me into her garden.

echoes of the past

november remembrance
of a time now long ago
when darkness was no stranger
at the house up on the hill
it came and had no mercy
playing havoc with our lives
it challenged us to somehow find
a way to stay together
through the pain of stormy years
a strange calm appeared to beckon
for all those years are history now
may they cease to smother the future
yet still it is a struggle
to leave the past behind
the wounds still fresh, as if to say
there remains some despair here
the thing about remembrance
you never do forget
the pain inside, the oceans cried
and how they brought us forward
for without the stranger of darkness
you never truly know
how bright the light which burns inside
shedding warmth on a love somehow shared
a love which is unconditional
even though it seems to hide
a love which wishes it could more freely flow
and speak what trembles inside . . .

Thirty-five: Gift of memory

"Onward to my destination, and nothing will stand in my way."
[MARTHA BONNER REID, 1987]

UP THE James Street steps, then right along the Mountain Brow: the city of Hamilton sprawled below me. I cut through the psychiatric hospital grounds, an almost sacrilegious act that engulfs me with a palpable peace. Despite the chaos and misery that permeates the sprawling structure, the irony of the calm does not escape me. It is eerie to seldom see a soul wandering about, for the tonic-like serenity of these well-tended grounds is beyond the trespass of those hidden inside. I pass by the circular buildings with the patchwork colour schemes and tinted windows, chilled by the sight of the wrought-iron bars. I feel an uncommon bond to this leper-like structure plunked on the edge of affluence on the west Hamilton Mountain. With each crossing, it is like reclaiming a part of the past on behalf of my Mom.

While Mom did eventually break free from those bars, ones both real and imagined, talking about the time she spent in that place has always been taboo. It is mentioned only when I'm chastised for taking that shortcut up to my parents' home from the downtown bus terminal. My Dad bitterly warns me that men escape all the time from "there" with relative ease, implying, of course, that those who do are a danger to society; by contrast, when Mom was in there, she was under lock and key.

Where once I heard only the anger in my Dad's admonishments, I am now aware of something far deeper. I see the pain in his eyes and hear the frustration in his voice. Although Mom echoes Dad's concerns for my safety when I traverse the grounds of her former residence, she does not betray the same anguish. With her recollection of that time now like dust, I still cannot help but wonder what particles of memory three decades on are evoked by that period of incarceration.

✳   ✳   ✳   ✳   ✳

For as long as I can remember, I become heavy-hearted whenever I happen upon homeless older women, or those who exhibit the telltale signs of a dispossessed psychiatric patient. When I lived for two years in Parkdale, the west-end Toronto neighbourhood with a high concentration of the like, not a day would go by that I would not cross paths with one of these overtly destitute souls. Yet no matter what part of the city I am in, time and again, I am haunted by the thought that any one of these women could have been my Mom. They pierce my consciousness and pervade my thoughts. I have given change, bought coffee, offered fruit, even garments of clothing. But seldom have I spoken, afraid of connecting with whatever is buried inside them, of knowing what obstacles have stood in their way, robbing them of a more fulfilling existence. Coming upon the "onward to my destination" affirmation Mom composed and included in a letter while I was travelling overseas, I cannot help but wonder whether she realized how much she had overcome to reach her destination of wellness.

[JANUARY 1997] Watching *Means of Grace*, a daughter's powerful and poignant documentary about her mother's ordeal with another mental illness: paranoid schizophrenia. I force myself to watch the part about electroshock. Slow tears give way to uncontrollable sobs as I heave against the back of the couch, my teeth clenched so tight the enamel grinds upon itself, as the woman's body contorts even moments after the wad of tissue is removed from her mouth. Sobbing for the tragedy of it all, my eyes squeezed shut so hard I see the same colours Mom must have as the electricity raced through her brain.

Yunee's tears console me, her arms a guardian angel-like wrap around my trembling body. My fears come spilling forth. There has been so much lost time. There remains so much I want to do for my Mom, yet somehow, I do nothing. I will never be able to handle the guilt and emptiness when she is gone. Days later, I replayed the electroshock segment over and over and over again, instilling in my brain the memory of it all; driven to vicariously experience what Mom did.

A deep-seated survival instinct gave my Mom the remarkable courage to weather two decades dogged by storms of depression, to tolerate an often emotionally abusive and psychologically damaging marriage, to carry on a life very much absent of her two offspring, to withstand a myriad of medications, and to stoically endure the near unspeakable horror of electroshock.

In the 1960s, the procedure for ECT was far from refined. Patients were given a mild sedative and an intramuscular relaxant to reduce the risk of bones dislocating or breaking during the minute-long seizure that was experienced after being jolted with anywhere from 70 to 175 volts of electricity. Because anesthetic was still not routinely administered, and the doses of relaxant and voltage were crudely calculated, abuses of treatment occurred. Granted, the techniques for ECT have been modified since the early 1960s. By the 1980s, when my Mom was subjected to her last series of treatments, the only obvious physical sign of shock passing through the body was betrayed by a slight trembling in the feet. It is the ethical element of ECT that remains. And for very legitimate reasons.

As a therapeutic practice, ECT boasts up to a 90% percent "success" rate for the treatment of severe depression, when administered to those who are not responding to antidepressants, have stopped eating and caring for themselves, and are at risk of dying or committing suicide. Proponents of ECT, who agree that the majority of patients will lose their short-term memory of events just prior to the treatment, are quick to point out that the impairment is temporary. Furthermore, they claim that any impediments of memory may be a symptom of the depression itself, as it affects the ability to concentrate and retain information. However, there is no shortage of research that indicates that some patients do lose portions of their memory permanently. This is particularly evident when a person is subjected to bilateral ECT over many years, as both short- and long-term memories are irretrievably damaged. There is no doubt in my mind that my Mom is a case in point of such brain damage, repeatedly finding herself at the mercy of doctors who were overtly indiscriminate in their repeated advocacy of shock treatments for her depressions.

For it was hundreds of those currents that stripped Mom of her memory, both short and long term. She has virtually no recollection of my brother Barry and me growing up. She was robbed of years no mother would ever willingly sacrifice. Sometimes, she will fake her ability to remember something, ashamed to admit, until I gently prod her, that in fact she does not. Several years ago, she began practicing "it must have slipped my mind," a more forgiving way of saying she forgot something in the everyday stream of things. When I put together two photo albums spanning the 1950s through the 1990s as a Christmas present for her in 1995, it was perhaps the greatest gift I could have ever given: the visual gift of memory.

In all fairness, the electroshock may not be solely to blame for her tattered memory. As Dr. Cove once explained, and I have experienced to some degree, the very nature of depression inhibits concentration, which in turn impairs memory, resulting in an amnesia-like effect. It is also quite possible Mom has learned to disassociate herself from the unpleasantness of the past, even as far back as her own childhood, teenage years, and wedding, well before the documented episodes of clinical depression began. In some ways, those voids in her memory are a blessing. They allow her to get on with her life and not be unduly plagued by the distress of frequent hospitalizations, miserable vacations, and constant, bitter quarrelling with my Dad. Periodically, Mom has asked whether she was ever mean to us kids. I've never been able to give her a straight answer, circling around it by reassuring her that I knew it was the illness, not she, that was responsible. I have a powerful need to protect her from the frightening, screaming mother she was at times.

Whereas Mom was defined by an illness for some twenty years, now the person that she is within identifies her. So long an introverted and almost subservient wife, Mom has found her voice, not in an aggressive way, but in a manner that is more assertive, and she is not as shy about expressing her opinion on different issues — even with Dad. In the words of one of her favourite Canadian contemporary singers, Burton Cummings, she is finally "Standing Tall." How vividly I remember attending a Burton Cummings concert at Hamilton Place with Mom in the late 1970s and the tears that glistened in her eyes when he belted out that trademark anthem. Two decades later, Mom has adopted it as one of her own.

Nevertheless, it is not lost on her, as she once commented to me, that Dad still tends to treat her as if she were sick. He remains quick to temper, has little patience for her chronic forgetfulness, or the internal clock by which she now moves in the world. So what if it takes her an hour to peel a few vegetables, three to clean the bathroom, or a full afternoon to compose a grocery list? At least she is doing things, and tasks are often extended, she admits, by her frequent wanderings over to a window to look for cardinals, blue jays, and rabbits, or perhaps even nothing at all. To her credit, Mom usually manages to rise above Dad's incessant chastising, accepting that he will likely never change, and does not let him bother her as she may have in the past. Perhaps the glass or two or three of wine a day helps her to cope with her matrimonial reality. She is not at all the same woman I worried would lose her way and relapse into depression when her lithium support group disbanded in the early 1990s. Somehow, it is a stronger and more confident woman who takes one day at a time. Not so much as a matter of choice, but of necessity. She cannot dwell on a past she barely remembers, nor worry about a tomorrow she will likely soon forget.

That Mom has not experienced an episode of clinical depression since 1982 continues to be a daily blessing. For years, I worried that certain life events would set my Mom over the edge again, not the least of which have included the upheaval following my father's job loss in 1984, the discovery of his affair in 1985, the disclosure of my homosexuality in 1992, and the two-year estrangement between Barry and me in the mid 1990s. Though each of those constituted a significant crisis, lithium prevented her from falling susceptible to a major depression.

Yet all the diamonds in the world cannot mask the dullness of her memory or the dimmed responsiveness of her emotions. ECT and drugs have trashed a significant portion of her mental functioning. By the time lithium entered her life at the age of 52, it could do no more than elevate her to a level of flatness. As much as she does not regress to the depths of despondency, neither does she demonstrate strong feelings of happiness. Her emotions are distressingly monotone, betraying the battered brain she now possesses. As her daughter, I feel cheated for lost time — ripped off. I feel greedy for wanting more than just her wellness. I selfishly want more than a mother on automatic pilot. I want a mother with whom I can converse at a level deeper than we do now. I want to be able to share more of my life without assuming she'll just forget so why bother telling her.

But that "why bother?" attitude is my self-defeatist streak, sprouted from the stoic independence I acquired as a child, that nothing I did or said really mattered. But it does matter. When Mom started on lithium, it was a time for her to start giving back to me. But I was not a very gracious receiver, for my more comfortable role as a giver had so long been established. It has taken me well into my thirties to appreciate that others, nobody more than my own mother, feel as good about giving as I do. My hand on the door, I now try to keep it open, never more to be forcefully closed. I welcome her to move freely through — or do I?

My perpetual homework is to accept the parameters of her fragmented memory and disaffected way of expressing emotions. She deserves to know what is happening in my life, for that life is worthwhile to her; it encompasses a meaning I can only venture to imagine. I resolve to start keeping notes about the little things to tell her, just as she does for me. Mom has always been a great note keeper. All around the house are little pieces of paper: in the laundry area, on the fridge, on her bedroom dresser, on the side of the sink, on the kitchen bulletin board, beside the phone. It is that pocket-sized memo pad beside the phone on which she jots down things to tell or ask me: Does our dog C.C. eat Dr. Ballard's food? If so, she has a coupon. Should she post my McMaster alumni mail, or keep it until I come next time? Do I use Carnaval-brand soap? She remembers she gave me a bar once, and if I liked it, she would pick some up — it was selling for 25 cents at Kresges, which was closing its doors for good. The trivial nature of our conversations betrays the simplistic way in which her mind works. Sometimes I wonder if it stopped developing when she gave birth to me. How many times I fight back tears of frustration for the emptiness of our communications, knowing it will never get better. I feel distant when we talk, and equally guilty when time passes and she ends up calling me first. For if the truth be known, were I simply to call and tell her I sharpened a pencil, she would be happy just to hear my voice.

Now time is slipping through my fingers. There is so much I want to do for her and say to her that I am paralyzed, muted by words and actions. Driven by a need to protect her, I can only fail miserably, overstepping the vague boundaries of what I can and cannot do for her. How could I have prevented her from tripping on the sidewalk, scraping her knees, spraining her wrists, and knocking our her front teeth when I was 40 miles away? How can I defend the timid way she orders a coffee at her favourite Tim Horton's, boldly asking for triple cream, then apologetically fumbling for change with her arthritic hands, frustrated by her own lack of deftness before an impatient cashier? How can I cover up the ingenuous, almost child-like way she questions repeatedly the pharmacist who prescribed antibiotics for a bee sting, if it is okay to take them with lithium and parnate? How do I reassure myself that at least she has the wherewithal to ask such critical questions? How do I ever find a way to stop overcompensating for what is not mine to control? For she is a study in contrasts: the innocence of youth and the wisdom of well-weathered years, juxtaposed in small but meaningful ways.

[CHRISTMAS DAY, 1994] With Dad downstairs, thankfully preoccupied by computer games, Mom stays with Yunee and me upstairs, where we talk and laugh over glasses of wine in the living room. When it comes time to make the turkey gravy, Yunee asks Mom for some tips. At first she is a little hesitant to be offering advice, not wanting it to seem as if she is telling us what to do. "Remove it from the heat while adding the flour. Keep stirring," she continues. It is something so trivial yet I feel proud that Mom knows how to do it. Suddenly she stops mid-sentence, apologizing for talking too much; this from a woman who has spent most of her life being told what to do and what not to do and who passed virtual years in bed without speaking. Now well into her sixties, the last thing she wants to be doing is imposing on others. Yet this is hardly a power struggle between three women. She is simply offering advice in her easygoing conversational way, not in a berating, condescending manner to which she and I have been so accustomed under my father's roof. I swallow hard. The moment conjures up vignettes of sadness. I choke back most of my tears. I give her a reassuring hug, knowing she cannot possibly talk too much after long years of silence.

✻   ✻   ✻   ✻   ✻

From the inside looking out, upon a bright sunny day. The circular room is silent, save for the low humming of the cold metal radiators. Stillness reigns, but for the gentle movement of the grey vertical blinds. Nothing seems to live here, not even the plants that hang from the rafters — merely artificial dust collectors. The trees outside stand naked, stark reminders of the season past; winter always the worst. But the passing sky is blue. The grass is turning greener; signs of spring regaining consciousness. On occasion a sparrow flits by. A forsythia bush prematurely blooms, pressing against the windows, trying to get in. Mocking the inmates crying to be free. A massive, misshapen tree stump sprouts dozens of healthy branches, a not-so-odd sighting here, just a random act of nature.

For here, the wards are scattered with such random acts. The world doesn't know they're in here; and if it did, would it care? For years I have walked across these grounds; now I too have crossed the line. Impossible to explain this logic to others, but then, they are not her daughter. Driven by a hunger to come full circle, to this home of tinted windows where she was locked behind the bars mere months after my birth — just another crazy person. The need to be here consoles me, for are we all not but random acts of nature?

not my mother

your shoulders droop, your gait robotic
your stare so vacant it chills
i search beyond your darkened eyes
hoping for a clue
where are you from, what traumas known
to render you like this
my eyes well up, my heart is heavy
why do i feel such pain
when women like you i see them
so listlessly on the street
the world rushes by, but no, not i
my sensitivity soars
for all intents and purposes
you could have been my mother
in and out of hospitals
she too has seen the depths
of cruel despair and darkened hours
when no one seemed to care
then like a miracle she was lifted
to heights for me unknown
on steady ground she lives her life
for now she's safe and sound

Thirty-six: The colour of joy

Maybe one day, Jann Arden's "Good Mother" and mine will meet ...

YEAR AFTER YEAR, Mom continues to be fine. For those who did not know her before lithium, she comes across so gentle, timid, so "reverent" my 93-year-old neighbour Impi once commented. I was pleased that someone pictured Mom that way: so fragile — afraid to trespass anyone, almost light-footed. Indeed, she carries herself like a mouse in a china shop. Thoughtful, genuine, caring, giving, and infinitely good-hearted: all typical of the words people use to describe her. She comes across as the calm in the midst of so many storms. The sentiments expressed in a 1997 birthday card from Renée Karsson, her neighbour of nearly 40 years, sum Mom up beautifully in my mind: *"It is an honour to know you Martha — you are one of the gentle souls in my life."*

Mom is a common sight on Bendamere Avenue, walking the four or five blocks down to the Garth Street bus stop, for she thinks nothing of taking public transit anywhere in the city. People often ask her, or wonder from their window, where on earth she is going all the time? Sometimes, she visits her elderly Aunt Edith, taking her a can of salmon for the sandwiches that are a coveted pleasure in the Macassa Lodge Nursing Home, where Edith resides. Or she may be off to meet her sister Iris or a friend for lunch. Otherwise, she is the happy wanderer, content to pass the day shopping, whether browsing, buying, or exchanging; walking for blocks; people-watching over a coffee and muffin — simple pleasures most cannot understand. But I do. How vividly I recall that day on the edge in September 1982, when she tearfully lamented to Dr. MacIntosh that all she wanted to be able to do was go look around the stores. She was not asking the world then; she never has and never will. After so many bedridden and hospital-ized days and weeks, she now has a firm grip on freedom, to touch the blue sky and claim the days for herself. No matter how tired she is or how many lithium years have passed, she recently confessed to me that she will never succumb to an afternoon nap, for fear she will not want to get up.

Once upon a time, I had not enough coloured pencils for the things Mom could not do when she was sick. Now, as the neatly packaged set of Laurentiens on my desk reminds me, all the coloured pencils in the world are hers to have and to hold, to colour the day in whichever shade she chooses.

[APRIL 1996] *Mournful creaking of the season's first swing, instills a feeling of loss within me; of emptiness for the times gone by; and for those which will never be.*

Ever the omnipotent child, I will always regret not fulfilling Mom's life with that elusive colour of joy: the gift of a grandchild. She remains on the outside looking in, always at photos of someone else's grandchildren. Admitting she had almost said "yes" when a stranger once asked if the infant she was holding was her granddaughter, when in fact it was her grandniece; overhearing her confess to a neighbour that she wishes she were indeed a grandmother. That I deny myself the rapture of motherhood is one thing; to deny Mom the coveted joy of grandmotherhood is quite another. Trapped by my past as a daughter, shaped by her dreams for herself, I wish I could offer her the chance to again hold the newborn flesh of her blood. But there will almost certainly be no christening of a new generation, for Barry and I share a common fear of passing on the depressive genes that are rooted in both our parents.

Instead, every November, Mom and I celebrate the birth of another year of her lithium life. I take her out for lunch or dinner and present her with a single red rose, silken or dried, for her corner table, where she has them all neatly arranged in an elegant china vase I bought when the roses numbered 10. Each slender stem is a testimony to her resilience, reminding me to be thankful for small miracles, like 25-cent bars of soap and gravy-making tips. That she may touch the blue sky forever.

baby's breath

though the November skies
breathe death among us
there is still the light
of rebirth
for while the baby's March breath
brought teardrops
the spirit now blooms
everlasting
with love Mom, for your courage to keep coming back . . .

Epilogue: Sobering thoughts

"The turning point in your life is some day you'd counted on to do the work you've never done. It doesn't come suddenly — you train yourself for it. It comes afer years and years of letting it run past you while you fretted yourself away."

[SAM SHEPARD as DASHIELL HAMMETT in *Dash and Lilly*]

[2003] IN MANY ways, I feel as if I have travelled a lifetime since beginning this book in March 1994. During the years that followed, in between cycles of depression and drinking, I somehow managed to create a manuscript worthy of the esteemed June Callwood's attention. In March 1999, I made the transition back into the paid workforce as a part-time employee of the Toronto Public Library. In May, that career all but came to a crashing halt. But by the grace of a force beyond me, I woke up this side of death following yet another destructive and poisonous drinking binge. Ghastly as that morning after was, it was a necessary evil, catapulting me straight to jail, no more passing "GO." I have been sober ever since, thanks to the extraordinary women of the Jean Tweed Centre.

To be sure, recovery has been the hardest and most important thing I have ever done for myself. How ironic — it was so frightfully difficult to be present and accounted for in my own life. And yet, recovery alone was not a panacea for clearing up the rubble of a past life, for cycles of depression kept recurring. In January 2001, still under the psychiatric care of Dr. Judith Cove, I began a course of antidepressant medication. Given that this is totally contradictory to my previously stated strong misgivings about medication, I debated as to whether or not I should "admit" to this turning of colour. But the whole point of this book is to write words that have too long dwelled in silence.

In March 2002, I turned 40. In November, my Mom and I celebrated the 20th year of her "wellness." Mid-way between those two landmarks, I met Althea Prince, Managing Editor of Women's Press. She has since become the self-described mid-wife on behalf of Women's Press, for the delivery of this, my first baby.

On a late January morning in 2003, I am writing this epilogue at a study carrel at an east-end branch of the Toronto Public Library. Coincidentally, I am at arm's length from books labelled with the spine numbers 616.8527: books about depression. Within mere months, my own book on the subject will join them.

The mid-day sun pours in through a window, drenching me with comforting warmth. I think back to the years of a past life, when I sought refuge from the chaos at home in the world of books at the Terryberry Library in my hometown. Now, at virtual middle age, it is as if I have come full circle. But these days, instead of running away from, I am travelling toward. I am consumed with unprecedented peace and calm. I have embraced a newfound love of the written word and the sharing of literary passion. I reflect upon a phrase from Virginia Woolf, who wrote in *The Waves*, "You cannot find peace in avoiding life." Tragically, she was consumed with being afraid of the day.

✻   ✻   ✻

That I have always been inclined to write has long been my bulwark against the blues. As a young girl, I remember waking early to the blessed quiet of Sunday mornings, trying to write short stories in the style of *Nancy Drew* or *Trixie Beldon* mysteries. But fiction did not come easy, for my head was blocked by a reality I could not express, only sought to escape. In the 1960s and 1970s when I was growing up, depression was a private illness. I believed we were the only family in the world experiencing it. Decades after Woolf's untimely death, the tragedy of mental illness and its ripple effect continue to destroy lives the world over at a staggering rate.

Thankfully, albeit slowly but surely, depression, and mental illness in general, are coming out of the closet and into memoirs, magazines, lecture halls, and onto television, the big screen, and billboards. Lives are being saved and salvaged in the process.

My Mom, Dad, brother, and I still do not openly talk about the years of my mother's depression and how they shaped us as a family. It is to our detriment that we allow the proverbial elephant to swallow up so much space in our lives. For better for worse, the writing of this book has been my way of talking.

Be not afraid of the day.

Without my journey,
And without the spring
I would have missed this dawn.

— SHIKI

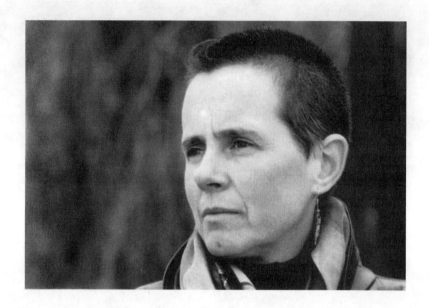

NANCY GRAHAM was born and raised in Hamilton, Ontario. She first wrote about mental illness in 1982, when she did a university research paper on electroconvulsive therapy. This fueled an interest in depressive disorders and their impact upon family dynamics. Graham's volunteer commitment is now focused on the work of the Jean Tweed Centre, a forerunner in the field of substance abuse treatment programs for women and their families in Ontario. She is the editor of the Centre's newsletter.

The author hopes that this book will offer some validation for others who have been affected by mental illness, and specifically clinical depression; that they may find her book waiting on a bookstore or library shelf, and know it was written for them.